THE OUTLIVE NATURAL REMEDIES BOOK

INSPIRED BY PETER ATTIA

THE ULTIMATE GUIDE TO MASTERING PETER ATTIA'S TEACHINGS

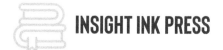

INSIGHT INK PRESS

© **Copyright 2024 by Insight Ink Press – All rights reserved.**

This document is geared towards providing exact and reliable information in regards to the topic and issue covered. The publication is sold with the idea that the publisher is not required to render accounting, officially permitted, or otherwise, qualified services. If advice is necessary, legal or professional, a practiced individual in the profession should be ordered.

From a Declaration of Principles which was accepted and approved by a Committee of the American Bar Association and a Committee of Publishers and Associations.

In no way is it legal to reproduce, duplicate, or transmit any part of this document in either electronic means or in printed format. Recording of this publication is strictly prohibited and any storage of this document is not allowed unless with written permission from the publisher. All rights reserved.

The information provided herein is stated to be truthful and consistent, in that any liability, in terms of inattention or otherwise, by any usage or abuse of any policies, processes, or directions contained within is the solitary and utter responsibility of the recipient reader. Under no circumstances will any legal responsibility or blame be held against the publisher for any reparation, damages, or monetary loss due to the information herein, either directly or indirectly.

Respective authors own all copyrights not held by the publisher. The information herein is offered for informational purposes solely, and is universal as so. The presentation of the information is without contract or any type of guarantee assurance.

The trademarks that are used are without any consent, and the publication of the trademark is without permission or backing by the trademark owner. All trademarks and brands within this book are for clarifying purposes only and are owned by the owners themselves, not affiliated with this document.

Disclaimer/Terms of Use
Product names, logos, brands, and other trademarks featured or referred to in this publication are the property of their respective trademark holders and are not affiliated with Knowledge Tree. The publisher and author make no representations or warranties with respect to the accuracy and completeness of these contents and disclaim all warranties such as warranties of fitness for a particular purpose. This guide is unofficial and unauthorized. It is not authorized, approved, licensed or endorsed by the original book's author or publisher and any of their licensees or affiliates.

All rights reserved. No portion of this book may be reproduced in any form without permission from the publisher, except as permitted by U.S. copyright law.

For permissions contact: edumasters.publishing@gmail.com
The Outlive Natural Remedies Book Inspired by Peter Attia, First Edition
ISBN: 979-8333477835
Written by: Insight Ink Press
Typesetting and text makeup by: Insight Ink Press

Printed in the United States of America

MAKE THE CHANGE,
NOT ONLY FOR YOURSELF

We believe that healing goes beyond the individual; it extends to the collective well-being of our communities and the world at large.

Your Purchase Supports a Greater Cause

With every purchase of this book, a meaningful portion of the proceeds will be donated to charitable organizations dedicated to health, wellness, and environmental sustainability. Your choice to embark on this journey of self-healing doesn't just benefit you; it also contributes to causes that align with the book's message.

Thank you for being a part of this meaningful endeavor. Together, we can create a world where self-healing is not just a personal journey but a collective movement for positive change. Your contribution matters, and we are deeply grateful for your support.

YOUR FREE GIFT

We wanted to take a moment to express our gratitude for your recent purchase from us. As a token of our appreciation, we are excited to offer you our best-selling workbook of Barbara O'Neill's Book "Self-Heal by Design".

To claim your free workbook, simply scan the QR code below with your smartphone or tablet, and follow the download instructions. This workbook are packed with valuable tips and exercises to help you start your self-healing journey and unlock the healthiest version of yourself.

In addition to the GIFT, you'll also have access to exclusive giveaways, discounts, and other valuable information.

TABLE OF CONTENTS

INTRODUCTION

In a world where the pursuit of well-being often involves navigating complex landscapes of modern medicine and lifestyle choices, the allure of natural remedies remains a constant beacon of wisdom. The Outlive Natural Remedies Book Inspired by Peter Attia's: The Ultimate Guide to Mastering Peter Attia's Teachings beckons readers to explore the profound teachings of Peter Attia in the context of holistic wellness.

This book is not just a compilation of remedies; it is a journey into the heart of holistic living, where mind, body, and spirit converge in a harmonious dance. Grounded in the foundational principles of natural healing, it seeks to unravel the innate healing power residing within each individual and illuminate the timeless connections between our well-being and the rhythms of nature.

As we embark on this enlightening expedition, readers are invited to rekindle their understanding of health, exploring the delicate balance between nutrition, hydration, sleep, and exercise. It transcends the mundane and dives deep into the therapeutic potential of foods, unveiling their healing power in fortifying the body's defenses, quelling inflammation, and sustaining cardiovascular harmony.

The narrative takes us into the realm of herbal medicine, where the bounty of nature's apothecary is explored. From understanding plant chemistry to creating effective herbal remedies, this book emphasizes the safety and efficacy of herbal treatments. Detoxification and cleansing are presented as essential practices for optimal wellness, while stress mastery unfolds as a symphony of well-being, harmonizing hormones and redefining our relationship with stress.

Beyond conventional approaches, the book introduces alternative therapies, inviting readers to consider chiropractic, physical therapies, homeopathy, and naturopathy as holistic avenues to well-being. Specialized topics, from managing chronic pain to nurturing heart health and navigating the challenges of cancer care, are approached with an integrative mindset, merging traditional wisdom with modern science.

This journey is not merely a theoretical exploration; it culminates in practical applications. Readers are encouraged to craft their personalized paths to natural wellness, assess their health mosaic, and set sail with personal health constellations. The book concludes with a crescendo of recipes designed for specific health conditions, reinforcing the idea that the kitchen can be a sanctuary for holistic healing.

In essence, The Outlive Natural Remedies Book is an invitation to rediscover the simplicity and effectiveness of natural remedies. It is a testament to the idea that true well-being is not a destination but a continuous journey—one that unfolds uniquely for each individual. Through the pages of this book, readers are empowered to embrace a holistic approach to health and embark on their own odyssey toward natural wellness.

ABOUT PETER ATTIA

Peter Attia is a prominent physician renowned for his pioneering work in the fields of longevity and health optimization. With a focus on the science of aging, nutrition, and preventive medicine, Attia has become a leading figure in the quest to extend human lifespan and improve the quality of life. His meticulous approach to health and wellness integrates cutting-edge research with practical, actionable advice, making his teachings accessible and impactful for a wide audience.

Peter Attia's journey in medicine began with an extensive educational background. He earned his medical degree from Stanford University, followed by a residency in general surgery at Johns Hopkins Hospital. His training also included a fellowship in surgical oncology at the National Cancer Institute, where he honed his skills and deepened his understanding of complex medical conditions.

Attia's professional path has been diverse, encompassing roles in both clinical practice and research. He has worked as a surgeon, a researcher, and a consultant, always driven by a relentless curiosity and a commitment to improving health outcomes. His experiences in these varied roles have given him a unique perspective on the interplay between medical interventions and lifestyle choices in achieving optimal health.

Peter Attia's primary focus is on longevity—the science of extending the human lifespan—and healthspan, the period of life spent in good health. He advocates for a comprehensive approach to health that includes nutrition, exercise, sleep, and stress management. His teachings emphasize the importance of understanding and mitigating the risks of chronic diseases such as cardiovascular disease, diabetes, and cancer, which are major contributors to mortality.

YOUR JOURNEY

These blank pages have been intentionally left empty to provide you with a space where you can reflect on your journey as you read through the book. Use this space to write down your goals, intentions, and aspirations for this journey. You can also take some time to reflect on your past experiences and how they have impacted your life.

By jotting down your thoughts and feelings, you will be able to compare your growth and progress at the end of this book.

CHAPTER 1:
UNEARTHING THE ABUNDANT VARIETY OF MEDICINAL FLORA

The realm of medicinal plants is a treasure trove of diversity, encompassing a vast array of species from every corner of the globe. These plants range from towering trees to delicate wildflowers, manifesting in various shapes, sizes, and habitats, each endowed with its unique set of healing properties. For millennia, cultures worldwide have relied on plants as medicine, seeking relief from ailments ranging from the common cold to chronic diseases. Whether cultivated in gardens, foraged from the wild, or passed down through traditional healing systems, medicinal plants offer a holistic approach to health and wellness, honoring the interconnectedness of the body, mind, and spirit.

Understanding the Healing Power of Plants

At the heart of herbalism lies an understanding of the intrinsic healing properties present in plants. From aromatic herbs that soothe the senses to potent botanicals with profound medicinal effects, plants harbor a wealth of bioactive compounds that contribute to their therapeutic value. Many medicinal plants are rich in vitamins, minerals, antioxidants, and other phytochemicals that support various aspects of health, including immune function, digestion, and circulation. Others possess specific pharmacological properties, making them effective remedies for particular ailments, such as anti-inflammatory, antimicrobial, and pain-relieving actions. By studying the unique chemical composition of plants and their interactions with the human body, herbalists unlock the healing potential of nature's pharmacy, harnessing the power of plants to promote health and vitality.

Bridging Tradition and Science in Herbal Medicine

Throughout history, diverse cultures have cultivated rich traditions of herbal medicine, passing down knowledge of medicinal plants through generations. Traditional systems like Traditional Chinese Medicine (TCM), Ayurveda, and Western Herbalism offer invaluable insights into the therapeutic properties and applications of herbs for health and healing. In addition to traditional practices, modern herbalism integrates scientific research and evidence-based approaches to validate the efficacy and safety of herbal remedies. Advances in botany, phytochemistry, and pharmacology illuminate the mechanisms behind herbal medicines, deepening our understanding of how plants exert their healing effects. Today, herbal medicine continues to evolve, with practitioners merging traditional wisdom with contemporary knowledge to craft effective, personalized treatment plans for those seeking natural alternatives to conventional medicine.

Herbalism as a Lifestyle: Cultivating a Deep Connection with Nature

Herbalism transcends mere healing; it embodies a way of life that fosters a profound connection with the natural world. By engaging with medicinal plants, herbalists cultivate a deep appreciation for nature's cycles, the earth's wisdom, and the interconnectedness of all living beings. Through the processes of growing, harvesting, and preparing herbs, herbalists develop reverence for plants and the ecosystems that support them. Attuned to nature's subtle rhythms, they observe changing seasons, lunar cycles, and the signs and signals of plants, fostering balance, vitality, and harmony within themselves and the world. Herbalism thus becomes a path not only to healing but also to personal growth, self-discovery, and ecological stewardship.

Proper plant identification is the cornerstone of safe and effective herbalism. With thousands of plant species in existence, accurate identification is critical to using plants for medicinal purposes. Mistaken identity can lead to serious consequences, including poisoning or adverse reactions. Herbalists must familiarize themselves with each plant's botanical characteristics, including leaves, flowers, stems, and roots. Consulting reliable botanical references, field guides, and experienced mentors helps confirm plant identities before harvesting or medicinal use.

Navigating Basic Botanical Terminology and Characteristics

Understanding fundamental botanical terminology and characteristics is essential for accurate plant identification. Key terms include:

- Leaf Arrangement: How leaves are arranged on a stem (e.g., opposite, alternate, whorled).
- Leaf Shape: The overall shape of a leaf (e.g., ovate, lanceolate, palmate).
- Leaf Margin: The edge of a leaf (e.g., serrated, toothed, entire).
- Leaf Venation: The pattern of veins on a leaf (e.g., pinnate, palmate).
- Flower Structure: The arrangement and composition of flowers (e.g., solitary, inflorescence, umbel).
- Fruit Type: The structure that develops from the ovary of a flower (e.g., berry, capsule, nut).

By mastering these concepts, herbalists can ensure they accurately identify and ethically harvest the plants they use, maintaining both their safety and the integrity of the ecosystems they interact with.

Different Ways of Practicing Ethical Wildcrafting and Foraging: Wildcrafting and foraging for medicinal herbs offer rewarding experiences, but responsible and ethical practices are essential. Here are some tips for ethical wildcrafting and foraging:

- Respect Nature: Harvest only what you need, leaving enough plants to ensure their survival and reproduction.
- Know the Law: Familiarize yourself with local regulations and restrictions on wildcrafting and foraging, including permits and protected species.
- Harvest Mindfully: Choose harvesting sites carefully, avoiding areas with pollution, pesticide use, or environmental hazards.
- Practice Leave-No-Trace: Minimize environmental impact by staying on designated trails, avoiding

trampling sensitive habitats, and packing out waste or litter.
- Express Gratitude: Show appreciation to plants, land, and ecosystems by offering prayers, blessings, or tokens of gratitude.

Adopting Sustainable Harvesting Practices: Sustainable harvesting practices are crucial for preserving wild plant populations and maintaining healthy ecosystems. Here are some guidelines for sustainable harvesting:

- Harvest Responsibly: Take only what you need, avoiding overharvesting from wild populations.
- Promote Regeneration: Harvest from abundant species, leaving mature plants, seeds, and plant parts for propagation.
- Support Biodiversity: Avoid harvesting rare or endangered species, prioritizing plants that are abundant and resilient.
- Rotate Harvesting Sites: Alternate harvesting locations to prevent depletion of plant populations in a single area.
- Monitor Impact: Regularly assess the health of harvested populations, adjusting practices as needed to minimize negative impacts.

Following these guidelines ensures herbalists' harvesting practices are sustainable, ethical, and respectful of the natural world.

How to Preserve the Potency of Herbs: Drying, storing, and preserving herbs are essential skills for any herbalist or home enthusiast seeking to extend their botanical treasures' shelf life and potency. Here's how to dry herbs using different methods:

- Air Drying: Air drying, one of the oldest and simplest methods, preserves herbs effectively. To air dry herbs, gather small bunches of freshly harvested herbs and tie them together with string or twine. Hang the bundles upside down in a warm, well-ventilated area away from direct sunlight. Allow the herbs to air dry until crisp and brittle, typically within 1 to 2 weeks, depending on humidity levels.
- Dehydrating: Using a food dehydrator for herb dehydration is convenient and efficient. Spread freshly harvested herbs in a single layer on dehydrator trays, setting the temperature to the appropriate setting for herbs (usually around 95°F to 115°F or 35°C to 46°C). Dehydrate herbs until thoroughly dried, typically 4 to 12 hours, depending on moisture content and thickness.
- Oven Drying: Oven drying offers another quick drying option, especially when time is limited. Spread herbs in a single layer on a baking sheet lined with parchment paper. Place the baking sheet in a preheated oven set to the lowest temperature (usually around 140°F or 60°C), leaving the oven door slightly ajar to allow moisture to escape. Check the herbs frequently, removing them once completely dry.

Ensuring Proper Handling and Storage: Preserving the potency of herbs extends beyond drying; proper handling and storage are equally critical. Here's how to ensure your dried herbs stay fresh and flavorful:

- Cooling and Cleaning: Let freshly harvested herbs cool completely before handling, as heat can cause wilting and loss of potency. Remove damaged or discolored leaves, gently brushing off dirt or debris.
- Storage Containers: Store dried herbs in airtight containers like glass jars, metal tins, or vacuum-sealed bags to shield them from moisture, light, and air. Label containers with the herb name and harvest date for freshness and potency.
- Storage Conditions: Keep dried herbs in a cool, dark place away from direct sunlight, heat sources, and humidity. A pantry, cupboard, or drawer provides the ideal environment for preserving flavor and potency.

Exploring Infusions, Blends, and Creative Preservation Ideas

Once dried and stored, there are countless ways to enjoy the benefits of herbs. Use dried herbs to create herbal infusions, blends, and mixtures for teas, culinary delights, bath products, and more. Get inventive and experiment with various herb combinations to discover unique flavors and therapeutic properties. With a touch of creativity, the possibilities for herbal preservation are endless.

With these techniques, you can ensure your herbs remain potent and flavorful, ready to be enjoyed whenever you need a taste of nature's healing bounty.

Crafting herbal infusions is a delightful journey into the realm of herbalism, offering a simple yet effective method to extract the medicinal properties and flavors of herbs. Follow these tips to create herbal infusions that soothe the soul and invigorate the senses:

- Steeping Process: When making herbal infusions, steep dried herbs in hot water for several minutes to unlock their medicinal properties and flavors fully.
- Straining Techniques: Once steeped, strain the infusion using a fine mesh strainer or cheesecloth to remove any residual herb particles, ensuring a smooth and clear liquid.
- Versatility in Usage: Enjoy the herbal infusion as a soothing tea or utilize it as a base for herbal remedies, culinary creations, and beauty products, expanding its versatility beyond a mere beverage.

Crafting Custom Herbal Blends: Experimentation is key when it comes to crafting custom herbal blends tailored to your preferences and needs. Here's how you can create unique herbal blends that cater to your specific requirements:

- Selecting Complementary Herbs: Combine different dried herbs based on their complementary flavors and therapeutic properties to achieve a harmonious blend that serves your intended purpose.
- Therapeutic Considerations: Blend herbs with specific therapeutic purposes in mind, whether it's for relaxation, digestion, immune support, or mood enhancement, ensuring that each blend serves a distinct health goal.
- Culinary Applications: Explore culinary applications for herbal blends by incorporating them into your favorite recipes, infusing dishes with layers of flavor and aromatic complexity.

Crafting Flavorful Herbal Mixtures: Crafting herbal mixtures opens up a world of possibilities for enhancing the taste and versatility of your culinary creations. Here are some creative ideas for crafting flavorful herbal mixtures.

- Fusion with Other Ingredients: Mix dried herbs with complementary ingredients such as salts, sugars, oils, or vinegars to create flavorful blends that elevate your cooking, seasoning, and preserving endeavors.
- Culinary Innovations: Experiment with different herbal mixtures in your culinary experiments, adding depth and dimension to dishes ranging from savory to sweet, and from appetizers to desserts.
- Preservation Techniques: Utilize herbal mixtures as a means of preserving seasonal herbs and extending their shelf life, ensuring that you can enjoy their flavors and benefits throughout the year.

Creative Ideas for Herbal Preservation

1. Crafting Herbal Vinegars:
- Infusion Process: Infuse dried herbs into vinegar to create flavorful herbal vinegars for both culinary

and medicinal applications. Simply place dried herbs in a glass jar, cover them with vinegar, and allow them to steep for several weeks to impart their essence into the vinegar.

- Versatile Applications: Once infused, herbal vinegars can be used in salad dressings, marinades, sauces, and vinaigrettes, adding a burst of herbal flavor to your culinary creations. Additionally, they can be utilized medicinally for digestive support, immune boosting, and overall wellness.

2. Crafting Herbal Oils:

- Infusion Technique: Infusing dried herbs into oil creates herbal oils that are not only flavorful but also versatile for culinary, massage, and skincare purposes. Fill a glass jar with dried herbs and cover them with a carrier oil such as olive oil or jojoba oil. Let the mixture steep in a warm, sunny spot for several weeks to allow the herbs to infuse their essence into the oil.
- Multi-Purpose Usage: Once infused, herbal oils can be used for cooking, adding a hint of herbal aroma and flavor to your dishes. They can also be used for massage, providing relaxation and nourishment to the skin. Additionally, herbal oils can be incorporated into skincare formulations, offering natural remedies for various skin conditions.

3. Crafting Herbal Butters:

- Flavorful Blending: Blend finely chopped dried herbs into softened butter to create flavorful and aromatic herbal butters. Mix and match herbs to suit your taste preferences and culinary applications, creating unique combinations that elevate your dishes.
- Culinary Enhancements: Herbal butters can be used as spreads for bread and crackers, toppings for grilled meats and vegetables, or flavorings for pasta and rice dishes. They add richness and complexity to your culinary creations, making them stand out with their unique herbal twist.

Essential Tools and Equipment for Herbal Preparation

Mortar and Pestle: A mortar and pestle offer timeless elegance and functionality in grinding herbs into powder or releasing their aromatic oils. These tools provide precise control over texture and consistency, essential for crafting herbal remedies, culinary delights, and aromatic blends.

Herb Grinder: An herb grinder proves invaluable for efficiently grinding larger quantities of herbs into fine particles. With sharp blades or teeth, it shreds herbs with ease, making them more manageable in recipes, infusions, and tinctures. An herb grinder ensures uniformity and ease of use in herbal preparations.

Kitchen Scale: Accuracy is paramount in herbal preparations, especially when measuring potent herbs and medicinal compounds. A kitchen scale offers precise measurements, ensuring consistency and precision in dosage and formulation. Whether crafting remedies or culinary creations, a kitchen scale is an indispensable tool for any herbal enthusiast.

Containers for Herbal Storage:

- Glass Jars: Glass jars provide ideal storage for dried herbs, herbal infusions, tinctures, and oils, offering airtight and light-resistant protection. They preserve the potency and freshness of herbs, ensuring their quality over extended periods. With glass jars, you can maintain the integrity of your herbal treasures with confidence.

- Airtight Containers: Airtight containers, such as metal tins or plastic containers with tight-fitting lids, safeguard dried herbs and herbal preparations from air, moisture, and light. They prevent degradation and loss of potency, ensuring that your herbal creations remain fresh and potent for longer durations.

- Herbal Sachets: Herbal sachets are charming pouches filled with dried herbs and aromatic botanicals, imparting natural fragrance to linens, drawers, and closets. They serve as delightful additions to herbal bath blends and potpourri, infusing your surroundings with the soothing scents of nature.

Equipment for Herbal Preparation:

- Strainers: Strainers play a vital role in separating liquid extracts from solid plant material in infusions, decoctions, and tinctures. Opt for strainers with fine mesh for thorough filtration, ensuring the purity and clarity of your herbal preparations.
- Cheesecloth: Versatile and indispensable, cheesecloth is commonly used for straining and filtering herbal extracts, oils, and infusions. It allows for thorough filtration while facilitating the easy passage of liquids, ensuring clarity and purity in your herbal creations.
- Funnel: A funnel simplifies the transfer of herbal preparations, oils, and tinctures into bottles and containers without spillage or waste. Look for funnels with wide mouths and narrow spouts for easy pouring and minimal mess. With a funnel, you can streamline your herbal preparation process with precision and ease.
- Dropper Bottles: Dropper bottles offer a convenient and controlled means of storing and dispensing liquid herbal extracts, tinctures, and essential oils. Equipped with dropper caps or pipettes, these bottles allow for precise dosage, making them ideal for oral or topical administration of herbal remedies. With dropper bottles, you can administer herbal extracts with confidence and accuracy.

Record your reflections, insights, and observations on the concepts discussed earlier.

Use this space to brainstorm, sketch, or jot down any questions that arise in your mind. Make it a truly personal experience.

CHAPTER 2:
PLANT CHEMISTRY: UNLOCKING NATURE'S PHARMACOPEIA

Understanding the intricate chemistry of plants is akin to unraveling the secrets of nature's pharmaceutical laboratory. Plants have evolved a remarkable array of chemical compounds, known as phytochemicals, each serving various functions from defense mechanisms against predators to attracting pollinators. However, it's their medicinal properties that truly capture our fascination. Among the diverse classes of phytochemicals, alkaloids, flavonoids, terpenes, phenols, and glycosides emerge as prominent players in the pharmacological theater unfolding within the plant kingdom.

Alkaloids: Nature's Potent Physiologists: Alkaloids are nitrogenous compounds found abundantly in plants, each exhibiting a unique set of physiological effects. These compounds, exemplified by morphine and caffeine, wield powerful influences on the human body, ranging from pain relief to central nervous system stimulation. Their diverse pharmacological actions make them invaluable assets in herbal medicine.

Morphine: The Pain-Relieving Powerhouse: Morphine, derived from the opium poppy, stands as one of nature's most potent analgesics. Its ability to alleviate pain and induce feelings of euphoria has made it a cornerstone in modern pain management and palliative care. Understanding the intricate mechanisms behind morphine's analgesic properties offers insights into novel approaches for pain relief and addiction treatment.

Caffeine: The Stimulating Substance: Caffeine, ubiquitous in coffee, tea, and various other plants, acts as a central nervous system stimulant, enhancing alertness and cognitive function. Its widespread use underscores its profound impact on human behavior and physiology. Delving deeper into caffeine's mechanisms of action sheds light on potential therapeutic applications beyond mere wakefulness promotion.

Quinine: A Tale of Malaria Treatment: Quinine, extracted from the bark of the cinchona tree, has long been revered for its antimalarial properties. Its discovery and subsequent use in treating malaria have saved countless lives throughout history. Exploring the chemical intricacies of quinine provides valuable insights into the development of novel antimalarial therapies and the fight against drug-resistant strains of the malaria parasite.

Flavonoids: Polyphenolic Powerhouses: Flavonoids, a diverse group of polyphenolic compounds, contribute to the vibrant colors of fruits, vegetables, and medicinal herbs. Beyond their aesthetic appeal, flavonoids boast a myriad of health-promoting properties, including antioxidant, anti-inflammatory, and immune-boosting effects. Their widespread distribution in the plant kingdom underscores their significance in human health and disease prevention.

Quercetin: Nature's Antioxidant Shield: Quercetin, abundant in foods like onions, apples, and berries, serves as a potent antioxidant, scavenging free radicals and protecting cells from oxidative damage. Its anti-inflammatory properties make it a promising candidate for managing conditions characterized by chronic inflammation, such as cardiovascular disease and arthritis.

Epigallocatechin Gallate (EGCG): Green Tea's Healing Elixir: EGCG, found predominantly in green tea, has garnered attention for its potent antioxidant and anticancer properties. Its ability to modulate cellular signaling pathways and inhibit tumor growth highlights its potential as a therapeutic agent in cancer prevention and treatment. Further exploration of EGCG's molecular mechanisms paves the way for the development of targeted cancer therapies.

Rutin: The Vascular Protector: Rutin, prevalent in citrus fruits, buckwheat, and tea, plays a crucial role in maintaining vascular health. Its ability to strengthen capillary walls and reduce inflammation makes it a valuable ally in the prevention and management of conditions such as varicose veins and hemorrhoids. Investigating rutin's vascular-protective mechanisms offers avenues for developing novel treatments for cardiovascular disorders.

Terpenes: Aromatic Allies of Well-Being: Terpenes, aromatic compounds responsible for the distinctive scents of plants, offer a treasure trove of therapeutic potential. From the calming aroma of lavender to the invigorating fragrance of eucalyptus, terpenes influence our senses and physiology in profound ways. Their antimicrobial, anti-inflammatory, and analgesic effects make them indispensable in essential oils and herbal remedies alike.

Linalool: Lavender's Soothing Scent: Linalool, abundant in lavender and several other aromatic plants, exerts anxiolytic and sedative effects, promoting relaxation and stress relief. Its ability to modulate neurotransmitter activity in the brain makes it a promising candidate for managing anxiety disorders and sleep disturbances. Exploring linalool's mechanisms of action unveils novel strategies for addressing mental health conditions.

Pinene: Pine's Respiratory Remedy: Pinene, prevalent in pine trees and coniferous plants, possesses bronchodilator and expectorant properties, making it beneficial for respiratory health. Its ability to alleviate symptoms of asthma and enhance airway clearance underscores its therapeutic potential in managing respiratory disorders. Investigating pinene's effects on airway smooth muscle relaxation offers insights into developing novel treatments for bronchospasm and airway obstruction.

Limonene: Citrus' Mood Lifter: Limonene, abundant in citrus fruits like lemons, oranges, and grapefruits, exhibits antidepressant and anxiolytic effects, enhancing mood and reducing stress. Its ability to modulate neurotransmitter levels in the brain makes it a promising candidate for managing mood disorders such as depression and anxiety. Exploring limonene's neuroprotective mechanisms offers avenues for developing novel antidepressant therapies.

Phenols: Guardians of Health and Vitality: Phenols, characterized by their aromatic ring structures and hydroxyl groups, showcase antioxidant properties that protect against oxidative stress and inflammation. Herbs like rosemary and sage are rich sources of these potent compounds, offering not only culinary flair but also a myriad of medicinal benefits. Phenolic compounds play a crucial role in fortifying the body against the detrimental effects of free radicals and inflammatory processes, thereby promoting longevity and vitality.

Rosmarinic Acid: Rosemary's Protective Powerhouse: Rosmarinic acid, abundant in rosemary and other aromatic herbs, exhibits antioxidant and anti-inflammatory properties, protecting cells from oxidative damage and reducing inflammation. Its potential in preventing and managing chronic diseases, such as cardiovascular disorders and neurodegenerative conditions, underscores its therapeutic significance. Investigating the molecular mechanisms of rosmarinic acid unveils opportunities for developing novel treatments targeting oxidative stress and inflammation.

Carnosic Acid: Sage's Neuroprotective Warrior: Carnosic acid, found predominantly in sage, demonstrates neuroprotective effects, safeguarding neurons from oxidative stress and age-related degeneration. Its ability to enhance cognitive function and memory retention holds promise for the prevention and treatment of neurodegenerative diseases like Alzheimer's and Parkinson's. Exploring carnosic acid's mechanisms of action offers insights into developing neuroprotective therapies to combat age-related cognitive decline.

Curcumin: Turmeric's Golden Healer: Curcumin, the bioactive compound in turmeric responsible for its vibrant color, possesses potent antioxidant and anti-inflammatory properties. Its ability to modulate signaling pathways involved in inflammation makes it a promising candidate for managing inflammatory conditions such as arthritis and inflammatory bowel disease. Investigating curcumin's therapeutic potential unveils novel strategies for combating chronic inflammation and associated diseases.

Glycosides: Sweet Solutions for Health: Glycosides, compounds in which a sugar molecule is bound to a non-sugar moiety, contribute to the pharmacological diversity of medicinal plants. From regulating heart function to aiding in bowel movements, glycosides offer a range of therapeutic benefits essential for human health.

Digitalis Glycosides: Foxglove's Cardiac Companion: Digitalis glycosides, derived from the foxglove plant, exert positive inotropic effects on the heart, increasing cardiac contractility and regulating heart rate. Their use in treating congestive heart failure and atrial fibrillation highlights their therapeutic significance in cardiovascular medicine. Exploring the pharmacokinetics of digitalis glycosides offers insights into optimizing their efficacy and safety in clinical practice.

Anthraquinone Glycosides: Senna's Bowel Buddy: Anthraquinone glycosides, abundant in plants like senna and rhubarb, exhibit laxative effects, promoting bowel movements and alleviating constipation. Their gentle yet effective action makes them a popular choice for relieving occasional digestive discomfort. Investigating the mechanisms of action of anthraquinone glycosides sheds light on their therapeutic potential and safety profile in managing gastrointestinal disorders.

Delving into the pharmacological intricacies of these bioactive compounds is very important. Each compound offers a unique set of therapeutic benefits, from pain relief and inflammation reduction to cognitive enhancement and mood stabilization. By elucidating the molecular mechanisms underlying their pharmacological actions, researchers and herbalists alike can harness the full potential of medicinal plants to formulate safe, effective, and personalized remedies tailored to individual needs. In this quest for knowledge and healing, the botanical world reveals itself as a boundless source of inspiration and innovation, holding the promise of a healthier, more vibrant future for humanity. Herbalists, with their deep understanding of plant medicine, wield an array of methods to prepare medicinal concoctions that harness the healing power of nature. Here's an exploration of some common methods, expanded to provide a comprehensive guide for those interested in the art and science of herbal medicine.

How to Make Infusions: Infusions gently coax out the soluble constituents of dried herbs by steeping them in hot water. This method is particularly effective for extracting the delicate and volatile components from plant parts like leaves and flowers. The process involves placing the herbs in a teapot or jar, pouring boiling water over them, and allowing them to steep for a specified period, usually between 5 to 15 minutes. This gentle method is ideal for preserving the integrity of volatile oils, flavonoids, and vitamins, which can be easily destroyed by prolonged exposure to heat.

Benefits and Uses of Herbal Infusions: Herbal infusions are versatile and can be used for various purposes:

- Therapeutic Teas: Infusions are often consumed as herbal teas, providing both medicinal benefits and a comforting experience. Common herbs used for therapeutic teas include chamomile for relaxation, peppermint for digestion, and elderflower for immune support.
- Culinary Uses: Infusions can also be used in culinary applications, such as flavoring broths, sauces, and desserts. For instance, lavender or rosemary infusions can add a unique flavor to dishes.
- Topical Applications: Infusions can be used as a base for skincare products, such as facial toners, hair rinses, and compresses for soothing skin irritations.

How to Prepare an Infusion:

- Select Your Herbs: Choose dried herbs, as fresh herbs may require a different preparation method.
- Measure: Use approximately 1 to 2 teaspoons of dried herbs per cup of water.
- Boil Water: Bring water to a boil and pour it over the herbs.
- Steep: Cover the container to prevent the escape of volatile oils and steep for the recommended time.
- Strain and Enjoy: Strain the herbs and enjoy the infusion hot or cold. Sweeten if desired with honey or another natural sweetener.

How to Prepare Decoctions: Decoctions involve a more robust approach, suitable for extracting the therapeutic compounds from tougher plant materials such as roots, bark, and seeds. This method involves boiling the plant material for an extended period, typically 20 to 45 minutes, to break down the fibrous components and release the medicinal properties.

- Benefits and Uses of Decoctions: Decoctions are highly concentrated and potent, making them suitable for addressing more severe or chronic conditions:
- Medical Treatments: Commonly used in traditional medicine systems, such as Traditional Chinese Medicine (TCM) and Ayurveda, decoctions are prescribed for a variety of ailments, including respiratory infections, digestive disorders, and inflammatory conditions.
- Nutrient Extraction: Decoctions are excellent for extracting minerals and other nutrients that may not be as readily available in infusions.

How to Prepare a Decoction:

- Select Your Herbs: Use dried or fresh roots, bark, or seeds.
- Measure: Use approximately 1 ounce of dried herb per quart of water.
- Simmer: Place the herbs in a pot, cover with cold water, and slowly bring to a boil. Reduce heat and simmer for 20 to 45 minutes.
- Strain and Store: Strain the herbs and store the decoction in a glass container. It can be kept in the refrigerator for up to three days.

Creating Potent Tinctures: Tinctures capture the essence of herbs in a potent liquid form through the use of solvents, such as glycerin or apple cider vinegar. This method involves macerating (soaking) the plant material in the solvent for several weeks to extract the medicinal compounds.

Benefits and Uses of Tinctures: Tinctures are highly concentrated and convenient for daily use:

- Long Shelf Life: Due to the alcohol content, tinctures can be stored for many years without losing their potency.
- Ease of Use: Tinctures are easy to dose, typically administered by dropperfuls, making them convenient for daily use or travel.
- Broad Applications: Tinctures can be used internally, added to water or juice, or applied topically for localized benefits.

How to Prepare a Tincture:

- Select Your Herbs: Fresh or dried herbs can be used. Fresh herbs are often preferred for their higher water content, which aids in extraction.

- Prepare the Herbs: Chop fresh herbs finely or use dried herbs as is.
- Choose a Solvent: You can use glycerin or apple cider vinegar can be used.
- Macerate: Place the herbs in a glass jar, cover them with the solvent, and seal them tightly. Shake daily and store in a dark place for 4 to 6 weeks.
- Strain and Bottle: Strain the mixture through a cheesecloth or fine mesh strainer and bottle the tincture. Label with the herb name and date.

Making Herbal Powders: Herbal powders involve grinding dried herbs into a fine consistency, making them versatile for various applications. This method is particularly useful for herbs that are difficult to extract using other methods.

Benefits and Uses of Herbal Powders: Herbal powders offer a convenient and versatile way to use herbs:
- Easy Dosing: Powders can be easily measured and added to foods, and beverages, or encapsulated for easy ingestion.
- Versatile Use: They can be incorporated into smoothies, sprinkled on food, or mixed into pastes and poultices for topical applications.
- Culinary Applications: Powders can be used to enhance the nutritional content of meals, such as adding turmeric powder to curries or smoothies.

How to Prepare Herbal Powders:
- Select Your Herbs: Ensure the herbs are completely dried to prevent mold growth.
- Grind: Use a mortar and pestle, coffee grinder, or dedicated herb grinder to pulverize the herbs into a fine powder.
- Sift: Sift the powder through a fine mesh sieve to ensure a uniform consistency.
- Store: Store the powder in airtight containers, away from light and moisture.

How to Prepare Herbal Oils and Salves: Herbal oils and salves extend the benefits of herbs to skincare and topical applications. Infusing carrier oils with herbs can create soothing and therapeutic preparations for various skin conditions.

Benefits and Uses of Herbal Oils and Salves: Herbal oils and salves provide localized relief and skin nourishment:
- Skincare: They are beneficial for moisturizing, soothing, and healing the skin. For example, calendula oil is known for its healing properties, while lavender oil is calming.
- Pain Relief: Herbal salves can be used to alleviate muscle pain, arthritis, and other inflammatory conditions.
- First Aid: Salves are effective for minor cuts, burns, and insect bites, providing both protection and healing.

How to Prepare Herbal Oils:
- Select Your Herbs: Use dried herbs to prevent spoilage.
- Choose a Carrier Oil: Common oils include olive oil, jojoba oil, and coconut oil.
- Infuse the Herbs: Place the herbs in a jar and cover them with the oil. Allow the mixture to infuse in a warm, sunny spot for 4 to 6 weeks, shaking occasionally.
- Strain and Store: Strain the oil and store it in a dark, cool place.

How to Prepare Herbal Salves:
- Prepare Herbal Oil: Follow the steps above to create an herbal oil.
- Melt Beeswax: In a double boiler, melt the beeswax.
- Combine: Add the infused herbal oil to the melted beeswax and stir well.
- Pour and Cool: Pour the mixture into jars or tins and allow it to cool and solidify.

Dosage and Administration Guidelines: Proper dosage and administration are crucial to ensuring the efficacy and safety of herbal remedies. The appropriate dosage varies based on several factors, including the herb's potency, the condition being treated, and individual patient characteristics such as age, weight, and overall health.

Factors Influencing Dosage: Herb Potency: Some herbs are more potent and require smaller doses, while others are milder and can be used in larger quantities.

Therapeutic Goals: Acute conditions may require higher doses for a shorter period, while chronic conditions often benefit from lower doses over an extended period.

Individual Characteristics: Age, weight, metabolism, and health status all influence the optimal dosage. Children and elderly individuals typically require lower doses.

Methods of Administration: Herbal remedies can be administered in various ways, each suited to different therapeutic needs:
- Internal Use: Includes infusions, decoctions, tinctures, and powders, which can be taken orally.
- Topical Use: Includes oils, salves, and poultices, which are applied directly to the skin.
- Inhalation: Essential oils and herbal steam inhalations are used for respiratory conditions.
- Baths: Herbal baths can provide both topical and systemic benefits through skin absorption and inhalation.

General Dosage Guidelines:
- Infusions and Decoctions: Typically, 1 cup (8 ounces) 2-3 times daily.
- Tinctures: Generally, 20-30 drops (about 1-2 milliliters) 2-3 times daily.
- Powders: Dosage varies depending on the herb and individual needs, usually 1-3 grams per day.
- Oils and Salves: Apply topically as needed, covering the affected area with a thin layer.
- Children and Elderly: Adjust dosage based on age, weight, and individual sensitivity, consulting a healthcare professional for guidance.

Monitoring and Adjusting Dosage:
- Start Low, Go Slow: Begin with the lowest effective dose and gradually increase as needed while monitoring for any adverse effects.
- Individual Response: Pay attention to how the body responds to the herbal remedy, adjusting the dosage accordingly.
- Interactions: Be aware of potential herb-drug interactions and adjust dosage or avoid combining certain herbs with medications.

Professional Guidance:
- Consultation: Seek guidance from a qualified herbalist, naturopathic doctor, or healthcare provider knowledgeable in herbal medicine.
- Personalized Recommendations: Receive personalized recommendations based on individual health history, current medications, and specific health goals.
- Follow-Up: Schedule follow-up appointments to assess progress, make any necessary adjustments, and ensure safety and efficacy.

By adhering to dosage and administration guidelines, individuals can maximize the benefits of herbal remedies while minimizing the risk of adverse effects, ensuring a safe and effective approach to natural healing.

Record your reflections, insights, and observations on the concepts discussed earlier.

Use this space to brainstorm, sketch, or jot down any questions that arise in your mind. Make it a truly personal experience.

CHAPTER 3:
EMBRACING THE FUNDAMENTALS OF HOLISTIC WELLNESS

Embark on an enlightening odyssey as we unravel the profound principles underpinning natural remedies, guided by the esteemed Barbara O'Neill. In the vast expanse of holistic health, the essence lies in the belief that our bodies possess an innate ability to heal. Join us as we journey through the Foundations of Health, where we explore the intricate tapestry of well-being.

The Innate Healing Power

At the core of natural remedies is the belief that the human body is a marvel, intricately designed for self-renewal. Envision these principles as the sturdy legs of a table, each contributing to the stability of the whole structure. As we delve into this chapter, we unravel the significance of nutrition, hydration, sleep, and exercise—pillars that, when nurtured, form a robust platform supporting the body's intrinsic healing processes.

Nutrition, often dubbed the building blocks of life, orchestrates good health. It is through the consumption of whole, unprocessed foods that the body receives the essential energy and nutrients needed for cellular processes, tissue repair, and the regulation of vital functions. The keystones of a healthful diet lie in the richness of antioxidants, vitamins, and minerals, acting as formidable guardians against the onslaught of diseases.

The importance of hydration cannot be overstated. Our bodies, predominantly composed of water, rely on this life-giving liquid for the efficient functioning of every system. Water acts as a purifier, flushing toxins, delivering nutrients to cells, and creating a moist environment for critical tissues. In its absence, the entire orchestration within the body falters, leaving us susceptible to a myriad of health issues.

Transitioning to the realm of rejuvenation, sleep emerges not merely as a passive state of rest but as a dynamic process of restoration and healing. As the body rests, it engages in the intricate dance of repairing muscles and tissues, consolidating memories, and releasing hormones crucial for growth and appetite regulation. Chronic sleep deprivation, an insidious disruptor, can pave the way for health maladies ranging from obesity to heart disease.

In the currency of health, exercise takes center stage—a dynamic investment that pays dividends in vitality. Strengthening the heart, improving circulation, toning muscles, and enhancing flexibility are but a few of its many returns. Regular physical activity stands as a formidable shield against chronic diseases, from heart disease to type 2 diabetes, while concurrently fostering mental well-being by unleashing endorphins that alleviate stress and elevate mood.

As we unfurl the layers of these foundations, witness the symbiotic relationship between them. Marvel at the interplay where good nutrition begets improved sleep, and hydration enhances the efficacy of exercise. Conversely, mismanagement of one element may trigger a domino effect, leading to a cascade of ill health.

This serves as a prelude to our immersive exploration into each component, where we unravel the scientific intricacies of their vitality. Join us as we equip ourselves with the knowledge to prevent, treat, and manage various diseases—not merely for longevity but to embrace a life teeming with vitality and vigor. The stage is set, and the journey awaits, promising a life sculpted by a well-nourished, well-rested, and well-exercised body.

UNRAVELING THE NUTRITIONAL TAPESTRY

Embark on a fascinating journey as we unravel the intricate layers of nutrition—a cornerstone in the mosaic of life. Beyond the mere act of eating, nutrition is a profound exploration of feeding every cell in your body the right way. This chapter serves as a gateway into the alchemy of ingredients that can transform our immunity, energize our days, and fortify our bones. Let us delve into the transformative power of nutrition, understanding how the quality of the fuel we provide our bodies shapes our overall health and wellness.

Nutrition, the alchemical science of nourishment, examines the profound relationship between diet and health. Essential nutrients—vitamins, minerals, fats, proteins, and carbohydrates—take center stage, each playing a unique role in maintaining optimal bodily function. Proteins, akin to the body's building materials, are deployed for the creation and repair of tissues. Carbohydrates stand as the primary energy source for all bodily functions, with the balance of complex carbs being crucial for sustained energy. Fats, often misunderstood, are essential for long-term energy storage, vitamin absorption, and cell membrane structure.

Macronutrients, the nutritional pillars needed in substantial amounts, include carbohydrates, proteins, and fats. Each serves a distinct purpose, highlighting the intricate dance within the body. Carbohydrates, the body's main energy source, require the right balance for sustained energy—found in complex carbs like whole grains and vegetables. Proteins, the body's building blocks, extend beyond meats and beans, thriving in nuts and select grains. Fats, the unsung heroes, are champions for brain health, energy, and hormone production, sourced from avocados, nuts, and fish to safeguard the heart and overall health.

While macronutrients bask in the spotlight, micronutrients—vitamins, minerals, and trace elements—play equally pivotal roles. These 'silent heroes' operate in small quantities, preventing disease, maintaining energy levels, and preserving skin and eye health. Explore the significance of vitamin D for bone health, antioxidants for cellular repair, and iron for blood oxygenation.

In the symphony of nutrition, water emerges as the forgotten yet most critical nutrient. Regulating body temperature, aiding digestion, and flushing out toxins, water acts as the solvent transporting nutrients to cells. Crucial for kidney function and maintaining electrolyte balance, water deserves its place as an indispensable player in the nutritional ensemble.

Beyond the mere act of consuming, nutrition intertwines with our lifestyle. Stress, sleep, and physical activity levels entwine with our dietary choices, shaping our overall health. Explore the profound interplay between diet and sleep, where poor nutrition can disrupt sleep, influencing dietary choices the following day.

As we journey forth, the importance of basing our diet on a variety of whole foods becomes apparent. Fruits, vegetables, whole grains, lean proteins, and healthy fats create a well-rounded diet foundational to a lifestyle promoting vitality and disease prevention. In the upcoming sections, we will navigate the application of these principles, crafting a personalized nutrition plan to support your health and well-being goals. The canvas is ready, and the brush poised for the artistry of a nourished, vibrant life.

NOURISHING THE ESSENCE: HYDRATION UNVEILED

Embark on a refreshing exploration as we delve into the life-sustaining act of hydration—a symphony of replenishment that goes beyond quenching thirst. Hydration, the essence of vitality, is more than a mere intake of water; it is a dynamic process ensuring every cell in your body functions at its zenith. Join us as we plunge into the depths of why hydration is a cornerstone of well-being, influencing physiological processes from circulation to temperature regulation.

Hydration, in its simplest form, is the act of keeping your body adequately supplied with water. This elixir is not merely a thirst-quencher; it is the lifeblood of every physiological process within your body. Comprising about 60% of your body, water is continuously utilized and must be replenished. The everyday actions of sweating, breathing, and waste elimination contribute to water loss, emphasizing the crucial need for replenishment. Failure to replace lost water can lead to dehydration, manifesting in mild symptoms like headaches and lethargy, or progressing to severe complications such as kidney stones and urinary tract infections.

The benefits of staying hydrated extend far beyond mere satisfaction. Adequate water intake lubricates joints, mitigating discomfort associated with wear and tear. It maintains a delicate balance of bodily fluids, playing a role in managing blood pressure and regulating heart rate. Hydration facilitates the seamless transportation of nutrients and oxygen to cells, ensuring your body operates at its peak efficiency, brimming with vitality.

The age-old adage of "eight glasses a day" serves as a foundational guideline, but individual hydration needs are nuanced, influenced by factors such as weight, climate, and activity level. A simple self-check involves monitoring the color of your urine—it should exhibit a light yellow hue, signaling optimal hydration. Dark urine, on the contrary, indicates a need for increased fluid intake.
Hydration isn't solely about water intake; it's a nuanced interplay with how your body utilizes water, influenced by diet and lifestyle. Factors such as high caffeine consumption can deplete hydration levels, as can diets rich in salty or sugary foods. On the flip side, incorporating water-rich foods like cucumbers, oranges, and strawberries into your diet becomes a delicious strategy to bolster hydration levels.

Maintaining optimal hydration isn't a one-size-fits-all endeavor; it's a personalized journey. It involves heeding the signals your body provides, understanding the impact of diet and lifestyle choices on hydration, and ensuring water is within arm's reach throughout your day. A seemingly simple step unfolds as a powerful catalyst for your overall well-being. Hydration—where simplicity meets profound impact.

WATER: THE VERSATILE LIFE FORCE

Embark on a journey into the realm of water—the body's most essential nutrient, a versatile key that unlocks the intricate mechanisms of life. Beyond being a mere thirst-quencher, water orchestrates a multitude of biological processes, a nurturing flow sustaining every cell in our microcosmic universe. Join us as we unravel the profound roles of water in the body, delving into the highways it constructs for transportation, the stages it sets for biochemical reactions, and the climate it regulates for temperature equilibrium.

Water is not merely a passive participant; it is the conductor of a ballet within our bodies. Acting as the medium for cellular activities, it orchestrates the transportation of life-giving oxygen and nutrients through blood and lymph fluid, while simultaneously whisking away the metabolic refuse. It stages biochemical reactions, actively participating as a reactant and serving as the solvent that dissolves and distributes vital compounds. In the intricate dance of bodily functions, water emerges as the linchpin.

Much like Earth's oceans control climate, water regulates our body temperature. It absorbs and redistributes heat, ensuring our internal environment remains conducive to optimal physiological function. Through this intricate dance, water becomes the guardian of our body's thermal equilibrium.

Joints glide seamlessly, cushioned by water-based fluids, while organs find refuge in moist membranes that protect and provide structure. Water emerges as the silent architect, enabling the grace of movement and safeguarding the delicate balance within our bodily architecture.

Staying well-hydrated parallels the harmonious flow of a river within its banks. The delicate balance ensures health by enhancing physical performance, boosting cognitive function, supporting digestion and weight management, aiding detoxification, and contributing to radiant skin health. It's a holistic approach, where the river of hydration reflects the vitality within.

Hydration is a personalized journey, not a one-size-fits-all recipe. The amount of water needed is influenced by age, weight, climate, activity level, and individual health conditions. Strategies for adequate hydration include heeding your body's signals, incorporating water-rich foods, monitoring indicators like clear urine, establishing hydration routines, and adding a touch of flavor to make the act enjoyable.

Hydration is more than a biological necessity; it is a cornerstone of a thriving body and mind. As we comprehend the profound role of water in our well-being, we unlock the potential to elevate our health to its highest tide. Drink up—the essence of vitality awaits in each sip, a simple yet profound act of nourishment seamlessly woven into the tapestry of daily life.

SLEEP: EMBRACING THE NATURAL HEALER

Embark on a journey into the often-overlooked realm of sleep—a cornerstone of the human health puzzle, intricately woven into the fabric of well-being. Beyond merely recharging energy, sleep unveils itself as a complex restorative process, a natural healer that supports cognitive function, emotional balance, and overall physical health. Join us as we unravel the multifaceted role of sleep, empowering ourselves to accord it the same respect bestowed upon diet and exercise.

The Silent Symphony of Sleep: Essential Roles Unveiled

Sleep, a silent symphony in the hustle of modern life, serves numerous vital functions, intricately choreographed for the benefit of our well-being:

- Cellular Repair and Growth: In the sanctuary of deep sleep, the growth hormone is released, facilitating cell repair and growth—a crucial process for recovering from the day's wear and tear.
- Cognitive Maintenance: Sleep becomes the custodian of memories, consolidating information and facilitating learning. Without adequate sleep, our cognitive abilities suffer, affecting focus, decision-making, and the acquisition of new knowledge.
- Metabolic Health: A regulator of hormones controlling appetite and insulin sensitivity, sleep plays a pivotal role in weight management and the prevention of diabetes.
- Emotional Regulation: Adequate sleep acts as a balancer of mood and emotions, reducing the risk of conditions like depression and anxiety.
- Immune System Function: A booster for the immune system, sleep becomes a defender against infections and holds implications for cancer prevention.

Sleep's Healing Power: A Panacea for Disease

In the context of disease, sleep's restorative power becomes even more pronounced, emerging as a potent ally in managing symptoms and improving outcomes:

- Cancer: Research suggests that quality sleep supports cancer treatments by maintaining a robust immune response and potentially slowing the growth rate of tumors.
- Heart Disease: Sleep influences blood pressure and cholesterol levels, crucial risk factors for heart disease. Quality sleep becomes a safeguard against these health threats.
- Diabetes: Proper sleep patterns regulate hormones affecting blood sugar levels, contributing to effective diabetes management.

Crafting a Sleep-Positive Environment: A Ritual of Well-Being

To harness the healing power of sleep, creating the right environment and adopting practices that promote restful sleep becomes imperative:

- Consistent Schedule: Establishing a consistent sleep schedule, going to bed and waking up at the same time every day, sets a rhythm for the body's internal clock.
- Sleep Hygiene: Keeping the bedroom dark, quiet, and cool signals to the body that it's time to wind down, creating a conducive atmosphere for rest.
- Pre-Sleep Routine: Engaging in relaxing activities before bed, such as reading or taking a warm bath, prepares the mind and body for rest.
- Diet and Exercise: Regular physical activity and a balanced diet enhance sleep quality. Timing is key—avoiding caffeine before bedtime and heavy meals contributes significantly.

Navigating Sleep Disorders: Natural Remedies for a Tranquil Night

Yet, achieving restorative sleep isn't always straightforward. Sleep disorders like insomnia, sleep apnea, and restless leg syndrome can disrupt this healing process. Natural remedies, such as valerian root, melatonin supplements, and magnesium, emerge as researched allies in the quest for better sleep.

Sleep's significance should weave through every chapter of a natural health guide, interacting with every aspect of well-being—from the food we eat to the stress we manage. By placing sleep at the center of a holistic health strategy, it becomes possible to enhance the efficacy of other natural remedies and lifestyle changes.

In summary, sleep transcends the notion of being a mere timeout from daily life. It unfolds as a state of intense biological activity, an underpinning force for health and healing capacities. By prioritizing and understanding sleep, we unlock its power as a natural healer—an ally in our quest for wellness and a vital component of any natural remedy plan. Embrace the essence of vitality that awaits in each restful night's sleep, for it is a journey toward profound well-being.

EXERCISE: UNLOCKING THE CURRENCY OF HEALTH

Embark on a journey into the transformative realm of exercise—an artful endeavor often hailed as one of the most effective ways to maintain and enhance health. Beyond the surface of burning calories and building muscle, exercise emerges as a transformative process, influencing the intricate workings of our body at a cellular level. Join us as we delve into the essence of exercise, dissecting it as the currency that fuels the economy of our body's health and impacts every facet of our well-being.

Picture your body as an economy, and exercise as its currency—a dynamic force that keeps the flow going, ensuring the seamless circulation of blood, nutrients, and vitality. It becomes an investment in the proper functioning of vital components, from the heart and lungs to muscles, brain, and mood.

The benefits of regular physical activity are profound, reaching far beyond the visible. Exercise becomes a shield against chronic diseases like heart disease, diabetes, and certain cancers. It serves as a weight management tool, a strengthener of bones and muscles, and a promoter of mental health and mood. Engaging in physical activity releases endorphins, the body's natural mood lifters, creating a cascade of positive well-being.

Moderate to vigorous exercise emerges as a powerful defender, boosting the immune system's defenses. For cardiovascular health, it enhances heart function, lowers blood pressure, and improves cholesterol profiles. It amplifies insulin sensitivity, a key player in diabetes management, contributing to effective blood sugar control.

In the realm of diseases like diabetes, heart conditions, and cancer, exercise transcends prevention—it becomes a complementary treatment. Beyond alleviating symptoms, it improves prognoses and enhances the overall quality of life. Cancer patients, for instance, experience improved fatigue, reduced anxiety, and boosted self-esteem through the transformative power of exercise.

Exercise isn't a one-size-fits-all prescription; it's a personalized journey. The key is to discover an activity that aligns with your lifestyle, interests, and health status. Whether it's walking, swimming, or weightlifting, the best exercise is the one that you'll consistently perform. Everyday activities, like gardening or taking the stairs, become valuable contributions to your exercise currency.

The path to exercise can be hindered by time constraints, lack of interest, or physical limitations. Creative solutions such as short workouts, finding an exercise buddy, or opting for low-impact exercises in the presence of joint pain become crucial in overcoming these barriers.

In conclusion, exercise stands tall as the cornerstone of a healthy lifestyle—a powerful tool accessible to virtually everyone. It adapts to individual needs and circumstances, offering a wealth of benefits. Like any currency, the more you invest in exercise, the richer you become in health. Embark on this journey, starting with small steps and gradually increasing activity, for it yields substantial health dividends over time. Exercise isn't just a physical endeavor; it's a journey toward vitality, enriching the currency of your health.

HOLISTIC HEALING RECIPES RELATED TO THIS CHAPTER

Vitality-Boosting Breakfast Bowl / Estimated Calories: 350 calories

Ingredients:
- 1 cup mixed berries (blueberries, strawberries, raspberries)
- 1/2 cup Greek yogurt
- 1/4 cup granola
- 1 tablespoon chia seeds
- 1 drizzle of honey

Instructions:
- Mix the berries and Greek yogurt in a bowl.
- Sprinkle granola and chia seeds on top.
- Drizzle honey for sweetness.

Hydrating Quinoa Salad / Estimated Calories: 400 calories

Ingredients:
- 1 cup cooked quinoa
- 1 cup cucumber, diced
- 1 cup cherry tomatoes, halved
- 1/2 cup feta cheese, crumbled
- 2 tablespoons olive oil
- Fresh basil leaves for garnish

Instructions:
- In a bowl, combine quinoa, cucumber, cherry tomatoes, and feta.
- Drizzle olive oil and toss gently.
- Garnish with fresh basil leaves.

Sleep-Inducing Warm Golden Milk / Estimated Calories: 100 calories

Ingredients:
- 1 cup almond milk
- 1 teaspoon turmeric
- 1/2 teaspoon cinnamon
- 1 teaspoon honey
- 1/4 teaspoon ginger (freshly grated)
- A pinch of black pepper

Instructions:
- Warm almond milk on the stove.

- Add turmeric, cinnamon, ginger, honey, and black pepper.
- Stir well and enjoy before bedtime.

Energizing Green Smoothie / Estimated Calories: 250 calories

Ingredients:
- 1 cup spinach
- 1/2 banana
- 1/2 cup pineapple chunks
- 1/2 cup Greek yogurt
- 1 tablespoon chia seeds
- 1 cup water or coconut water

Instructions:
Blend all ingredients until smooth.
Pour into a glass and garnish with chia seeds.

Exercise-Fueling Chicken and Quinoa Bowl / Estimated Calories: 450 calories

Ingredients:
- 4 oz grilled chicken breast, sliced
- 1 cup cooked quinoa
- 1 cup mixed vegetables (broccoli, bell peppers, carrots)
- 1 tablespoon olive oil
- Lemon juice for flavor

Instructions:
- Sauté the mixed vegetables in olive oil.
- Assemble the bowl with quinoa, grilled chicken, and sautéed vegetables.
- Squeeze lemon juice for freshness.

Remember, these are just rough estimates, and actual calorie counts may vary. Adjust portion sizes according to your dietary needs and goals. Enjoy these recipes as part of your holistic approach to health!

Record your reflections, insights, and observations on the concepts discussed earlier.

Use this space to brainstorm, sketch, or jot down any questions that arise in your mind. Make it a truly personal experience.

CHAPTER 4:
NOURISHING WITH PURPOSE
THE HEALING POWER OF FOODS

Embark on a captivating and enlightening exploration into the profound healing potential of foods—an age-old concept now intricately intertwined with modern scientific research. This chapter unveils the transformative impact of a carefully curated diet, demonstrating how certain foods can serve as potent tools in preventing, alleviating, and even reversing various medical conditions. Join us on this comprehensive journey, shedding light on the medicinal properties of foods that transcend their role as mere sustenance.

Superfoods for Immunity: Fortifying the Body's Defenders

Delve deeper into the intricate network of the immune system, a complex web of cells and proteins that stand as the body's staunch defender against infections. Unveil the power of superfoods, an illustrious category encompassing not only the well-known citrus fruits like grapefruits, oranges, and lemons but also the unsung heroes such as red bell peppers, broccoli, garlic, ginger, spinach, and yogurt. These superfoods deliver a concentrated arsenal of vitamins, minerals, and antioxidants that fortify the immune system, offering a natural defense against pathogens. Explore how the synergistic combination of these nutrients creates a resilient shield, enhancing the body's ability to ward off illnesses.

Anti-Inflammatory Foods: Quelling the Flames of Chronic Inflammation

Chronic inflammation, a silent contributor to numerous health conditions ranging from heart disease to arthritis and Alzheimer's, finds its foil in a diet rich in anti-inflammatory foods. Embark on a journey through the omega-3 fatty acids found in the succulent flesh of salmon and the tiny but mighty flaxseed. Delve into the lycopene-rich realms of tomatoes, savor the golden elixir of olive oil, and embrace the vibrant greens of spinach, kale, and collards. These foods orchestrate a symphony of relief, reducing inflammation and safeguarding against the ravages of chronic health issues. Uncover the intricate biochemical dance between these foods and the body's inflammatory response, painting a vivid picture of how mindful dietary choices can positively impact overall well-being.

Foods That Fight Cancer: A Nutrient Shield Against Cellular Damage

Certain foods emerge as true champions in the fight against cancer, armed with a diverse array of antioxidants and phytochemicals. Journey through the cruciferous realm of broccoli and Brussels sprouts, recognizing their rich content of glucosinolates, which studies suggest may play a pivotal role in reducing the risk of cancer. Savor the antioxidant-rich bounty of berries, each tiny jewel protecting cells from free-radical damage associated with cancer. Delight in the beta-carotene-laden carrots and their potential to reduce rates of certain types of cancer, including stomach cancer. Discover the protective fiber found in beans and whole grains, a shield against colorectal cancer. These foods become a potent nutrient shield, defending cells from damage and potentially preventing the formation of cancer. Navigate through the intricacies of how these foods interact with cellular processes, providing insights into their cancer-fighting potential.

Heart-Healthy Foods: Sustaining Cardiovascular Harmony

The cardiovascular system, a vital component of the body's intricate machinery, requires careful maintenance for longevity and well-being. Navigate the expansive landscape of heart-healthy foods, each playing a unique role in sustaining cardiovascular harmony. Encounter the soluble fiber found in the humble oats, a dietary hero that helps lower cholesterol levels by binding to it in the digestive system and removing it from the body. Revel in the antioxidant-rich bounty of berries, with their potential to protect blood vessels and promote heart health. Delve into the creamy goodness of avocados, a source of healthy fats that can contribute to managing cholesterol levels. Explore the omega-3-rich treasures of salmon and mackerel, proven to lower triglycerides and blood pressure. Uncover the nutritional richness of nuts and seeds, containing omega-3s, fiber, and vitamin E, which collectively contribute to lowering the risk of heart disease. These heart-healthy foods become invaluable allies in maintaining healthy blood vessels and a steady heartbeat, reducing the risk of heart disease and stroke. Dive into the intricate biochemical processes through which these foods impact cardiovascular health, gaining a deeper understanding of their role in sustaining this vital system.

HOLISTIC HEALING RECIPES RELATED TO THIS CHAPTER

Immune-Boosting Citrus Salad / Estimated Calories: 200 calories

Ingredients:
- 1 cup mixed citrus fruits (grapefruits, oranges, lemons)
- 1/2 cup red bell peppers, diced
- 1/2 cup broccoli florets
- 1 clove garlic, minced
- 1 tablespoon fresh ginger, grated
- 1 cup spinach leaves
- 1/2 cup Greek yogurt (as dressing)

Instructions:
- Combine citrus fruits, red bell peppers, broccoli, garlic, and ginger in a bowl.
- Toss in fresh spinach leaves.
- Drizzle with Greek yogurt for a creamy, immune-boosting dressing.

Omega-3 Rich Salmon Delight / Estimated Calories: 400 calories

Ingredients:
- 6 oz grilled salmon fillet
- 1 tablespoon flaxseed (sprinkled on top)
- 1 cup kale, sautéed in olive oil
- 1 cup cherry tomatoes, halved
- Lemon wedges for flavor

Instructions:
- Grill the salmon until cooked.
- Sauté kale in olive oil until wilted.
- Assemble the plate with grilled salmon, sautéed kale, cherry tomatoes, and sprinkle flaxseed.
- Squeeze lemon wedges for freshness.

Cancer-Fighting Berry Smoothie Bowl / Estimated Calories: 250 calories

Ingredients:
- 1 cup mixed berries (blueberries, strawberries, raspberries)
- 1/2 cup broccoli florets (frozen for a thicker texture)
- 1 tablespoon chia seeds
- 1/2 cup carrot juice
- 1/2 cup Greek yogurt

Instructions:
- Blend berries, broccoli, chia seeds, carrot juice, and Greek yogurt until smooth.
- Pour into a bowl and top with additional berries.

Heart-Healthy Avocado Oatmeal / Estimated Calories: 350 calories

Ingredients:
- 1/2 cup oats, cooked
- 1/2 avocado, sliced
- 1/4 cup mixed berries
- 1 tablespoon mixed nuts and seeds (walnuts, almonds, chia seeds)
- Honey for sweetness

Instructions:
- Cook oats according to package instructions.
- Top with sliced avocado, mixed berries, and nuts/seeds.
- Drizzle with honey for added sweetness.

Anti-Inflammatory Tomato Basil Pasta / Estimated Calories: 400 calories

Ingredients:
- 2 cups whole grain or gluten-free pasta
- 1 cup cherry tomatoes, halved
- 1/4 cup olive oil
- 2 cloves garlic, minced
- 1/2 cup fresh basil, chopped

- Salt and pepper to taste

Instructions:
- Cook pasta according to package instructions.
- In a pan, sauté garlic in olive oil until fragrant.
- Add cherry tomatoes and cook until they soften.
- Toss cooked pasta with the tomato mixture and fresh basil.
- Season with salt and pepper.

Fiber-Rich Bean and Quinoa Salad / Estimated Calories: 350 calories

Ingredients:
- 1 cup cooked quinoa
- 1 cup mixed beans (black beans, chickpeas, kidney beans)
- 1/2 cup cherry tomatoes, quartered
- 1/4 cup red onion, finely chopped
- 2 tablespoons olive oil
- Fresh cilantro for garnish

Instructions:
- Combine cooked quinoa, mixed beans, cherry tomatoes, and red onion in a bowl.
- Drizzle olive oil and toss gently.
- Garnish with fresh cilantro.

Cancer-Fighting Grilled Veggie Skewers / Estimated Calories: 300 calories

Ingredients:
- 1 zucchini, sliced
- 1 eggplant, cubed
- 1 bell pepper, diced
- 1 red onion, sliced
- 8 cherry tomatoes
- 1 tablespoon olive oil
- Lemon juice for flavor

Instructions:
- Thread zucchini, eggplant, bell pepper, red onion, and cherry tomatoes onto skewers.
- Brush with olive oil and grill until vegetables are tender.
- Squeeze lemon juice before serving.

Heart-Healthy Mackerel Salad / Estimated Calories: 250 calories

Ingredients:
- 1 can (4 oz) mackerel, drained
- 2 cups mixed greens
- 1/2 cucumber, sliced
- 1/4 cup cherry tomatoes, halved
- 1 tablespoon olive oil
- Balsamic vinegar for dressing

Instructions:
- Combine mackerel, mixed greens, cucumber, and cherry tomatoes in a bowl.
- Drizzle with olive oil and balsamic vinegar.

Feel free to experiment with these recipes, adjusting ingredients and flavors to suit your taste preferences. The key is to enjoy delicious meals that also contribute to your overall well-being. Happy cooking!

Record your reflections, insights, and observations on the concepts discussed earlier.

Use this space to brainstorm, sketch, or jot down any questions that arise in your mind. Make it a truly personal experience.

CHAPTER 5:
HARNESSING NATURE'S APOTHECARY - HERBAL MEDICINE

Embark on a fascinating journey through the realms of herbal medicine, a practice deeply rooted in ancient wisdom and now experiencing a resurgence in popularity. Also known as phytotherapy, herbal medicine employs plants and their extracts to foster health and combat illnesses. As we delve into this time-honored tradition, discover the origins, evolution, and modern acceptance of herbal medicine, unlocking the potent healing potential found in every leaf, root, flower, and berry.

Travel back in time to unravel the historical tapestry of herbal medicine, tracing its roots through ancient civilizations in Egypt, China, and India. Explore how these cultures documented the use of plants for medicinal purposes, forming the cornerstone of traditional healing practices. Witness the evolution of herbal medicine, where every part of a plant becomes a healing ally, whether consumed directly, brewed into teas, or transformed into tinctures, capsules, and powders. Gain insights into the belief that plants house natural substances capable of promoting health and alleviating illness, creating a bridge between ancient wisdom and contemporary healthcare.

Witness the harmonious convergence of traditional herbal wisdom with modern scientific recognition. Delve into a growing body of research that isolates active compounds in plants, unveiling their medicinal properties. Explore examples like digoxin, a heart medication derived from the foxglove plant, showcasing how herbal knowledge seamlessly integrates into conventional healthcare. As herbal medicine gains acknowledgment and acceptance in modern science, trace its journey from ancient traditions to becoming an integral part of contemporary healthcare practices.

Common Herbs and Uses: Nature's Medicinal Arsenal

Embark on a journey through well-known herbs, each offering unique benefits to health and wellness. Explore the anti-nausea properties of ginger, the anti-inflammatory and antioxidant effects of turmeric, the cognitive function-enhancing capabilities of Ginkgo Biloba, and the immune-boosting powers of Echinacea. Delve into the vast herbal landscape, discovering how these botanical allies contribute to well-being and provide holistic support for various conditions.

Uncover the tailored solutions herbal medicine offers for specific health conditions. For cancer support, explore the potential of turmeric and green tea, harnessing their antioxidant properties. For heart health, discover the benefits of hawthorn and garlic in supporting cardiovascular function. In the realm of diabetes, explore how cinnamon and fenugreek may aid in regulating blood sugar levels. While acknowledging the effectiveness of herbal remedies, navigate the importance of cautious use, especially for those with pre-existing conditions or undergoing specific medical treatments.

Recognize the supportive role herbs play in cancer care, understanding their potential to boost the immune system, alleviate side effects of conventional treatments, and improve overall quality of life. Explore the anti-inflammatory properties of turmeric (Curcumin), the nausea-alleviating benefits of ginger, and the liver-protective qualities attributed to Milk Thistle. Acknowledge that while herbs are not a cure for cancer, they can complement conventional treatments, contributing to a more holistic and supportive approach to cancer care.

Embark on a journey through herbs that contribute to a heart-healthy lifestyle. Uncover the potential of hawthorn in improving circulation and lowering blood pressure. Delve into the cholesterol-lowering effects of garlic and the omega-3 fatty acids found in flaxseed, beneficial for heart health. Explore how these herbs become integral components of cardiovascular wellness, managing blood pressure, reducing cholesterol levels, and supporting overall heart health.

Explore the realm of herbs that show promise in helping regulate blood sugar levels, crucial for managing diabetes and prediabetes. Delve into the potential of cinnamon to lower blood sugar levels, the glycemic control benefits of fenugreek, and the sugar-craving reduction and blood sugar level-lowering capabilities of Gymnema Sylvestre. Acknowledge these herbal allies as valuable components in the dietary management of diabetes, understanding their role in promoting balanced blood sugar levels.

Safety and Efficacy of Herbal Remedies: Navigating the Herbal Landscape with Care

While nature's remedies offer a rich tapestry of options for health and wellness, it's essential to approach herbal medicine with care. Navigate the safety considerations, consulting healthcare providers before starting any herbal regimen, particularly for those with existing health conditions or taking medications. Emphasize the importance of choosing high-quality products from reputable sources to ensure purity and potency. Stay vigilant about potential side effects and interactions with other medications, fostering a balanced approach that integrates traditional wisdom with contemporary scientific standards.

Dive into the nuanced realm of herbal medicine safety, recognizing that while herbs are natural, they are not universally safe for everyone. Emphasize the importance of consulting healthcare professionals, choosing high-quality products, and being aware of potential side effects and interactions. Understand that the efficacy of herbal remedies can vary, and while traditional wisdom often guides their use, ongoing scientific research contributes to evidence-based information. Approach herbal medicine with an open mind and a critical eye, recognizing its potential as a valuable addition to one's health regimen.

In conclusion, herbal medicine offers a rich tapestry of options for supporting health and treating illnesses. As research continues to unfold, the integration of these natural remedies into mainstream healthcare provides a more holistic approach to disease prevention and management. The chapter emphasizes the paramount importance of safety and informed use, highlighting that with careful consideration and professional guidance, herbs can become valuable additions to one's health regimen. The intricate dance between traditional wisdom and contemporary standards paves the way for a harmonious symphony of healing, where herbs become indispensable allies in the pursuit of vibrant health and well-being.

HOLISTIC HEALING RECIPES RELATED TO THIS CHAPTER

Anti-Inflammatory Turmeric and Ginger Tea / Estimated Calories: 10 calories

Ingredients:
- 1 teaspoon turmeric powder
- 1 teaspoon grated fresh ginger
- 1 teaspoon honey
- 1 cup hot water

Instructions:
- Mix turmeric, ginger, and honey in hot water.
- Steep for 5 minutes, strain, and enjoy.

Heart-Healthy Garlic and Herb Roasted Salmon / Estimated Calories: 300 calories

Ingredients:
- 2 salmon fillets
- 3 cloves garlic, minced
- 1 tablespoon olive oil
- 1 teaspoon dried thyme
- Salt and pepper to taste

Instructions:
- Preheat oven to 400°F (200°C).
- Mix garlic, olive oil, thyme, salt, and pepper.
- Rub the mixture over salmon fillets.
- Roast for 15-20 minutes or until salmon flakes easily.

Diabetes-Friendly Cinnamon and Fenugreek Oatmeal / Estimated Calories: 250 calories

Ingredients:
- 1/2 cup rolled oats
- 1/2 teaspoon ground cinnamon
- 1/4 teaspoon ground fenugreek
- 1 cup almond milk
- Berries for topping

Instructions:
- Cook oats with almond milk, cinnamon, and fenugreek.
- Top with berries before serving.

Immune-Boosting Echinacea and Citrus Salad / Estimated Calories: 150 calories

Ingredients:
- Mixed greens
- 1 orange, peeled and sliced

- 1/2 grapefruit, peeled and segmented
- 1 teaspoon echinacea tincture (optional)
- Olive oil and balsamic vinegar for dressing

Instructions:
- Arrange mixed greens, orange slices, and grapefruit segments.
- Mix olive oil, balsamic vinegar, and echinacea for dressing.

Ginkgo Biloba and Blueberry Smoothie / Estimated Calories: 200 calories

Ingredients:
- 1 cup blueberries (fresh or frozen)
- 1/2 banana
- 1/2 cup Greek yogurt
- 1 teaspoon Ginkgo Biloba powder
- Honey to taste

Instructions:
- Blend blueberries, banana, Greek yogurt, and Ginkgo Biloba powder until smooth.
- Sweeten with honey as desired.

Cancer-Fighting Broccoli and Kale Stir-Fry / Estimated Calories: 120 calories

Ingredients:
- 2 cups broccoli florets
- 1 cup kale, chopped
- 1 tablespoon olive oil
- 2 cloves garlic, minced
- 1 teaspoon soy sauce

Instructions:
- Stir-fry broccoli and kale in olive oil until tender.
- Add minced garlic and soy sauce.
- Cook for an additional 2 minutes.

Hawthorn Berry and Apple Compote / Estimated Calories: 90 calories

Ingredients:
- 2 apples, peeled and diced
- 1/2 cup hawthorn berries
- 1 tablespoon honey
- 1/2 teaspoon cinnamon

Instructions:
- Simmer apples, hawthorn berries, honey, and cinnamon until apples are soft.
- Mash slightly for a compote texture.

Remember to consider your individual health needs and consult with a healthcare professional before incorporating herbs into your diet, especially if you have pre-existing conditions or are on medications. Enjoy these herbal-infused delights on your path to well-being!

Record your reflections, insights, and observations on the concepts discussed earlier.

Use this space to brainstorm, sketch, or jot down any questions that arise in your mind. Make it a truly personal experience.

CHAPTER 6:
PURIFYING THE BODY: DETOXIFICATION AND CLEANSING FOR OPTIMAL WELLNESS

In the intricate tapestry of modern life, our bodies find themselves entwined with an assortment of toxins, a consequence of our surroundings and the additives that sneak into our daily nourishment. This continuous exposure to unwanted elements can accumulate within, potentially laying the groundwork for health concerns over time.

Beyond being a fleeting health trend, detoxification emerges as a harmonious biological response embedded in the intricate dance of our bodily processes. While our bodies inherently engage in detoxification daily, the intensified exposure to toxins in the contemporary era can strain these natural systems. Detoxification steps in as a guardian, nurturing the body's natural processes and ushering in a cascade of benefits:
- Amplifying the body's innate detoxification systems.
- Elevating energy levels and fostering mental clarity.
- Fortifying immune function.
- Enhancing digestion and championing gut health.
- Championing overall wellness and erecting barriers against potential diseases.
- Diverse Vistas of Detoxification: A Multifaceted Approach

Detoxification methods weave a diverse tapestry, each thread aiming to alleviate the burdensome weight of toxins on the body. The canvas includes:

- Fasting: A strategic pause from regular food intake, offering the digestive system respite and aiding in the graceful departure of toxins.
- Juice Cleanses: An immersion in the vibrant hues of fruit and vegetable juices, a nutrient-rich elixir that fuels the body while encouraging the elegant art of detoxification.
- Water Therapy: Imbibing increased volumes of water, sometimes infused with the botanical symphony of herbs or fruits, orchestrating a cleansing melody within.
- Sweating: A symphony of saunas and physical exertion, encouraging toxins to waltz out through the pores.

- Colon Cleansing: A meticulous choreography involving enemas or colonic irrigation, choreographed to cleanse the colon and elevate digestive health.
- Feasting on Detoxifying Elixirs: The Symphony of Nutrient-Rich Foods

Delight in the symphony of detoxifying foods, each note playing a crucial role in bolstering the body's natural detoxification processes:

- Leafy Greens: Enter the verdant realm of spinach, kale, and chlorophyll-rich greens, cleansing companions for the body.
- Cruciferous Vegetables: A ballet of broccoli, cauliflower, and Brussels sprouts, supporting the liver's choreography of detoxification.
- Fruits: Dance with the antioxidant-rich rhythm of berries, apples, and citrus fruits, harmonizing in fiber to facilitate toxin removal.
- Garlic and Onions: The sultry tango of sulfur compounds, partnering with the liver in the intricate art of detoxification.
- Green Tea: Immerse in the antioxidant-rich ambiance of green tea, a conductor orchestrating detoxification while enhancing liver function.

Crafting Your Personal Detoxification Symphony: Programs and Protocols

The orchestration of detox programs and protocols unfolds with a myriad of choices, each presenting a unique melody. Considerations for a symphonic detox program include:

- Duration: The duration of the detox journey, ranging from a brief interlude to an immersive symphony lasting several weeks.
- Dietary Guidelines: An exquisite arrangement emphasizing organic, whole foods while extinguishing the discordant notes of processed foods, sugars, and alcohol.
- Supplemental Support: Enhance the symphony with supplements like milk thistle or dandelion root, fortifying the liver's role in this grand composition.
- Lifestyle Changes: Join the dance of stress reduction, improved sleep, and the rhythmic beats of regular exercise, integral components of the detoxification symphony.

HOLISTIC HEALING RECIPES RELATED TO THIS CHAPTER

Verdant Detox Salad / Estimated Calories: 300 calories

Ingredients:
- 2 cups spinach (washed)
- 1 cup kale (chopped)
- 1 cucumber (sliced)
- 1 avocado (diced)
- 1 tablespoon chia seeds
- Lemon-tahini dressing (lemon juice, tahini, olive oil, salt, and pepper)

Instructions:
- Toss spinach, kale, cucumber, and avocado in a bowl.
- Sprinkle chia seeds on top.
- Drizzle with lemon-tahini dressing.

Cruciferous Symphony Stir-Fry / Estimated Calories: 200 calories

Ingredients:
- 1 cup broccoli florets
- 1 cup cauliflower florets
- 1 cup Brussels sprouts (halved)
- 2 tablespoons coconut oil
- Garlic and ginger (minced)
- Tamari sauce (to taste)

Instructions:
- Stir-fry broccoli, cauliflower, and Brussels sprouts in coconut oil.
- Add minced garlic and ginger.
- Season with tamari sauce.

Berry Citrus Infusion / Estimated Calories: 20 calories

Ingredients:
- 1 cup mixed berries (strawberries, blueberries, raspberries)
- 1 orange (sliced)
- Mint leaves
- 1 liter water

Instructions:
- Combine berries, orange slices, and mint in a pitcher.
- Fill with water and let it infuse for a few hours.

Garlic-Ginger Detox Elixir / Estimated Calories: 10 calories

Ingredients:
- 1-inch ginger (sliced)
- 2 garlic cloves (minced)
- Juice of 1 lemon
- 1 tablespoon honey
- 2 cups hot water

Instructions:
- Steep ginger and garlic in hot water for 5 minutes.
- Add lemon juice and honey.

Green Tea Bliss Smoothie / Estimated Calories: 150 calories

Ingredients:
- 1 cup brewed green tea (cooled)
- 1 cup kale (stems removed)
- 1 frozen banana
- 1/2 cup pineapple chunks
- Chia seeds (for garnish)

Instructions:
- Blend green tea, kale, frozen banana, and pineapple until smooth.
- Pour into a glass and sprinkle chia seeds on top.

Citrus Burst Detox Water / Estimated Calories: 10 calories

Ingredients:
- 1 lemon (sliced)
- 1 lime (sliced)
- 1 orange (sliced)
- Fresh mint leaves
- 2 liters water

Instructions:
- Combine lemon, lime, orange slices, and mint in a large pitcher.
- Fill with water and refrigerate for a refreshing detox water.

Feel free to customize these recipes based on your taste preferences and dietary needs. These refreshing and nutrient-packed options can be delightful additions to your detoxification symphony. Enjoy the culinary exploration of nourishing your body!

Record your reflections, insights, and observations on the concepts discussed earlier.

Use this space to brainstorm, sketch, or jot down any questions that arise in your mind. Make it a truly personal experience.

CHAPTER 7:
THE ART OF STRESS MASTERY: A SYMPHONY OF WELL-BEING

In the intricate symphony of life, stress emerges as a persistent note, weaving itself into our daily existence. Yet, the resonance it carries can significantly influence our health and well-being. Chronic stress, akin to a somber undertone, has been intricately linked to an array of diseases, ranging from the solemn echoes of heart ailments and diabetes to the shadows cast by mental health disorders. To unravel the profound secrets of well-being, it becomes paramount to dissect the role stress plays in orchestrating the dynamics of disease and cultivate a rich repertoire of effective stress management techniques.

Stress, particularly when it assumes a persistent presence, unravels its intricate chaos within our physiological and psychological realms. It sets off a hormonal cascade, unleashing the powerful duo of cortisol and adrenaline, orchestrating the body for a "fight or flight" response. While this physiological dance proves beneficial in acute situations, its persistent performance becomes a maestro conducting detrimental effects across various bodily systems. The prolonged crescendo of stress has been intricately linked to a compromised immune system, an elevated risk of cardiovascular diseases, the exacerbation of pre-existing conditions like asthma, and the haunting specters of mental health issues such as anxiety and depression.

Crafting Harmony Through Natural Stress Relief Strategies

The symphony of stress management unfolds as a melodic blend of lifestyle changes and natural techniques, presenting a vibrant palette for cultivating well-being:

Physical Activity: The rhythmic cadence of regular exercise emerges as a powerful stress buster, not only releasing the euphoric notes of endorphins but also harmonizing the body for a night of restful sleep—a sanctuary often disrupted by the dissonance of stress.

Healthy Diet: The gastronomic maestro guides us through a balanced diet adorned with antioxidants and essential nutrients, leading the body through the harmonious coping of stress. Foods rich in magnesium, omega-3 fatty acids, and vitamin C become virtuoso notes in the composition of stress reduction.

Adequate Sleep: Within the harmonious realm of stress management, good sleep hygiene takes center stage. Establishing a regular sleep routine, abstaining from caffeine and screens before bedtime, and creating a sanctuary of relaxation contribute to the crescendo of improved sleep quality.

Social Support: A network of friends and family forms the backdrop, providing emotional support and a sense of belonging—a sanctuary for coping with the harmonies of stress.

The delicate composition of relaxation techniques unfolds, each movement contributing to the harmony of stress relief:

Deep Breathing: A simple yet powerful movement, deep breathing emerges as a crescendo, activating the body's relaxation response. Techniques such as diaphragmatic breathing add depth to the composition, focusing on filling the abdomen rather than the chest with air.

Progressive Muscle Relaxation: A rhythmic dance of tension and release traverses different muscle groups, reducing physical tension and mental anxiety in a mesmerizing cadence.

Guided Imagery: A visual tapestry unfolds, involving the mind in picturing serene scenes or a series of experiences—a movement that shifts the focus away from stress.

Harmonizing Hormones: A Prelude to Balance

The chronic saga of stress can disrupt the hormonal equilibrium, leading to a dissonance of fatigue, weight gain, and mood disorders. The symphony of natural hormone balance includes:

Regular Exercise: A conductor in the hormonal orchestra, regulating insulin and cortisol, contributing to the rhythmic flow of well-being.

Healthy Fats: Incorporating avocados, nuts, and seeds composes a soothing melody, supporting hormone production in the body's symphony.

Reducing Sugar and Refined Carbs: An allegro of caution, avoiding these elements harmonizes the insulin and hormonal cadence.

Stress Management Practices: The activities of meditation and yoga join the hormonal composition, a chorus contributing to the reduction of cortisol levels.

Adequate Sleep: In the nocturnal movement of well-being, sleep plays a pivotal role in regulating various hormones, including growth hormone and cortisol.

Expanding our exploration of stress management, let us delve deeper into an encore of techniques that further enrich the symphony of well-being:

Art and Creativity: Channeling the creative energies becomes an expressive movement, offering a therapeutic outlet for stress release. Engaging in artistic pursuits, be it painting, or writing, provides a canvas for emotional expression and release.

Nature Therapy: Stepping into the natural tapestry of the outdoors becomes a restorative interlude. Nature therapy, whether through forest bathing, hiking, or simply basking in green surroundings, offers a harmonious escape from the cacophony of daily stressors.

Laughter Therapy: Embracing the infectious laughter becomes a therapeutic crescendo. Laughter, whether through comedy, socializing, or engaging in activities that tickle the funny bone, releases endorphins and fosters a light-hearted perspective.

Journaling: Unleashing the power of words becomes a cathartic movement. Journaling allows the exploration of thoughts and emotions, providing clarity and insight into the sources of stress and avenues for resolution.

Technology Detox: A rhythmic pause from the digital symphony becomes essential. Disconnecting from constant notifications and screens for designated periods allows the mind to rejuvenate and reclaim a sense of balance.

Harvesting the Fruits of Stress Management

By weaving this comprehensive array of stress management techniques into the intricate tapestry of our lives, we embark on a journey not only to diminish the harmful effects of stress but to elevate the entire composition of our health and quality of life. The realization dawns that managing stress is not about eradicating it entirely; rather, it is about mastering the art of responding to it in a healthier and more harmonious way.

The symphony of well-being encompasses not just the absence of stress but the presence of a resonant and vibrant melody, echoing through the corridors of our lives. As we conduct this grand orchestra, let us celebrate the diversity of movements, each contributing to the harmonious dance of health and vitality. The art of stress mastery unfolds not as a mere chapter but as a perpetual symphony, with each note playing a crucial role in the grand composition of our well-being.

HOLISTIC HEALING RECIPES RELATED TO THIS CHAPTER

Harmonious Salad Symphony / Calories: Balanced and nutrient-packed, approximately 400 calories per serving.

Ingredients:
- Mixed greens (rich in antioxidants)
- Avocado (healthy fats)
- Walnuts (omega-3 fatty acids)
- Berries (vitamin C)
- Grilled chicken (lean protein)

Instructions:
- Toss the mixed greens with sliced avocado, walnuts, berries, and grilled chicken.
- Drizzle with a light vinaigrette made with olive oil and citrus for an extra burst of antioxidants.

Zen Quinoa Bowl / Calories: Around 450 calories, offering a perfect balance of nutrients.

Ingredients:
- Quinoa (protein and magnesium)
- Salmon (omega-3 fatty acids)
- Spinach (iron and relaxation)

- Cherry tomatoes (vitamin C)

Instructions:
- Cook quinoa and top with grilled salmon, sautéed spinach, and cherry tomatoes. Season with herbs and a squeeze of lemon for a delightful, stress-busting bowl.

Relaxation Smoothie / Calories: Approximately 250 calories, a refreshing and energizing treat.

Ingredients:
- Banana (potassium)
- Greek yogurt (protein)
- Berries (antioxidants)
- Chia seeds (omega-3 fatty acids)

Instructions:
- Blend banana, Greek yogurt, berries, and chia seeds for a creamy and nutritious smoothie.
- Sip slowly, savoring each sip for a moment of calm.

Tranquil Sleep Elixir / Calories: Virtually zero, promoting relaxation without adding to your daily intake.

Ingredients:
- Chamomile tea
- Lavender honey
- Sleep-inducing herbs (valerian root, passionflower)

Instructions:
- Brew a cup of chamomile tea, add a spoon of lavender honey, and infuse with sleep-inducing herbs.
- Sip this elixir before bedtime for a restful night's sleep.

Creative Energy Stir-Fry / Calories: Approximately 350 calories, a delicious and artistic way to nourish the body.

Ingredients:
- Colorful vegetables (bell peppers, broccoli, carrots)
- Tofu or lean protein of choice
- Sesame oil (healthy fats)

Instructions:
- Stir-fry vibrant vegetables and tofu in sesame oil.
- The burst of colors and flavors stimulates creativity while providing essential nutrients.

Remember, the essence of these recipes lies not just in the calories but in the harmony they bring to your well-being. Enjoy these dishes as part of your symphony for a healthier and more vibrant life!

Record your reflections, insights, and observations on the concepts discussed earlier.

Use this space to brainstorm, sketch, or jot down any questions that arise in your mind. Make it a truly personal experience.

CHAPTER 8:
EXPLORING ALTERNATIVE THERAPIES:
A HOLISTIC JOURNEY
TO WELL-BEING

Delving into the realm of alternative therapies invites us into a world of healing practices that stand outside the conventional boundaries of Western medicine. Rooted in holistic principles, these therapies transcend the mere alleviation of symptoms, aiming to treat the entire individual—body, mind, and spirit. Rather than directly combating illness, they seek to harmonize the body's natural healing mechanisms, offering a unique approach to health and well-being.

Acupuncture, a jewel in the crown of traditional Chinese medicine, involves the strategic insertion of ultra-thin needles at specific points on the body, known as acupuncture points. This practice is believed to rebalance the flow of energy (Qi) within the body. While Western scientists hypothesize that it may stimulate nerves, muscles, and connective tissue, triggering the body's natural painkillers and enhancing blood flow.

In the same holistic vein, acupressure, a close relative to acupuncture, foregoes needles and relies on the application of pressure to specific points using fingers, palms, elbows, or specialized devices. Grounded in the same principles as acupuncture, acupressure seeks to stimulate the body's innate self-curative abilities. Widely used for pain management, stress reduction, and overall well-being, acupressure provides a non-invasive pathway to holistic health.

Chiropractic and Physical Therapies: Aligning Body and Mind

Chiropractic care zeroes in on disorders of the musculoskeletal system and the nervous system, recognizing their impact on overall health. Through hands-on spinal manipulation and alternative treatments, chiropractors strive to restore proper alignment, particularly in the spine, fostering the body's ability to heal without resorting to surgery or medication. This manipulation aims to rejuvenate mobility in joints constrained by tissue injuries.

Complementing chiropractic care, physical therapies encompass a spectrum of techniques employing movements and manipulative therapies to enhance function and alleviate pain. Exercises, stretching, massage, and the application of modalities such as ultrasound or hot and cold therapy form part of this holistic approach. The overarching goal is to improve mobility, alleviate pain, and enhance overall fitness and health.

Homeopathy and Naturopathy: Harnessing Nature's Remedies

Homeopathy embraces the principle of "like cures like," utilizing infinitesimal amounts of natural substances—plants and minerals—to stimulate the healing process. Rooted in the belief that substance-inducing symptoms in a healthy person can, in minute doses, treat those same symptoms in illness, homeopathy offers an unconventional avenue for healing.

Naturopathy, or naturopathic medicine, delves into a realm of alternative practices often branded as "natural" and "self-healing." Embracing pseudoscientific approaches such as homeopathy, herbalism, and acupuncture, alongside dietary and lifestyle counseling, naturopathy presents a comprehensive yet alternative approach to health.

Harmony in Diversity: A Holistic Pursuit of Health and Wellness

Each of these alternative therapies brings forth a unique perspective on health and healing, often serving as complements to conventional medical treatments. Embracing a holistic paradigm, they underscore the significance of treating the entire person—mind, body, and spirit—for the attainment of optimal health and wellness.

While the scientific backing varies among these therapies, their common goal unites them: to facilitate healing and enhance quality of life through a holistic, non-invasive approach. As individuals embark on the exploration of alternative therapies, it remains crucial to seek guidance from healthcare professionals, especially when navigating existing health conditions or concurrent medication use.

Expanding Horizons: The Ongoing Evolution of Alternative Therapies

The landscape of alternative therapies is continually evolving, with emerging modalities gaining recognition. As the tapestry of alternative therapies unfolds, individuals are empowered to explore diverse avenues for holistic well-being. While some modalities may resonate more strongly with certain individuals, the overarching theme remains rooted in the holistic approach to health—acknowledging the interconnectedness of mind, body, and spirit.

In conclusion, the exploration of alternative therapies extends beyond the boundaries of conventional medicine, embracing a holistic canvas that acknowledges the intricate interplay of physical, mental, and spiritual elements in the pursuit of well-being. While the efficacy and acceptance of these therapies may vary, their presence in the evolving landscape of health and wellness highlights the ongoing quest for diverse and holistic approaches to healing.

As individuals navigate this expansive terrain, seeking balance and harmony, the importance of collaboration with healthcare professionals cannot be overstated. Whether integrating alternative therapies into an existing healthcare regimen or exploring them as standalone practices, informed and collaborative decision-making ensures a holistic and comprehensive approach to well-being. The journey toward health and vitality is a tapestry woven with threads of diversity, each alternative therapy contributing a unique hue to the ever-evolving masterpiece of holistic well-being.

HOLISTIC HEALING RECIPES RELATED TO THIS CHAPTER

Qi-Boosting Tea Infusion

Ingredients:
- Green tea (antioxidant-rich base)
- Ginger (anti-inflammatory)
- Honey (natural sweetness)
- Lemon (vitamin C boost)

Instructions:
- Brew a cup of green tea, add a few slices of ginger, a teaspoon of honey, and a squeeze of lemon.
- This infusion aims to harmonize energy flow, providing a soothing and revitalizing experience.

Calories: Minimal, around 10-20 calories, offering a refreshing beverage for holistic well-being.

Acupressure Stress-Relief Snack

Ingredients:
- Almonds (magnesium-rich)
- Dark chocolate (antioxidant)
- Dried cherries (anti-inflammatory)

Instructions:
- Create a mix of almonds, dark chocolate chunks, and dried cherries.
- Enjoy this acupressure-friendly snack to promote stress relief and boost mood.

Calories: Balanced, around 150-200 calories per serving, a guilt-free delight for mind and body.

Chiropractic Alignment Smoothie Bowl

Ingredients:
- Greek yogurt (protein)
- Pineapple (anti-inflammatory)
- Spinach (iron and relaxation)
- Chia seeds (omega-3 fatty acids)

Instructions:
- Blend Greek yogurt with pineapple and spinach.
- Top with chia seeds for a chiropractic-inspired smoothie bowl that promotes overall alignment and well-being.

Calories: Approximately 300 calories, a nutrient-packed bowl for a harmonious start to the day.

Homeopathic Healing Soup

Ingredients:
- Bone broth (collagen for joint health)
- Turmeric (anti-inflammatory)

- Garlic (immune-boosting)
- Lentils (protein)

Instructions:
- Simmer bone broth with turmeric, garlic, and lentils.
- This homeopathic-inspired soup aims to support overall healing and well-being.

Calories: Nourishing and hearty, around 250 calories per serving.

Naturopathic Wellness Salad

Ingredients:
- Kale (nutrient-rich base)
- Quinoa (protein)
- Berries (antioxidants)
- Avocado (healthy fats)

Instructions:
- Toss kale, quinoa, berries, and avocado for a naturopathic-inspired salad.
- Drizzle with a lemon vinaigrette for a refreshing and holistic approach to wellness.

Calories: Balanced and nutrient-packed, approximately 350 calories per serving.

Remember, these recipes are not just about the ingredients but the intention behind them—harmony, balance, and holistic well-being. Enjoy these culinary creations as part of your journey towards a healthier and more harmonious life!

Record your reflections, insights, and observations on the concepts discussed earlier.

Use this space to brainstorm, sketch, or jot down any questions that arise in your mind. Make it a truly personal experience.

CHAPTER 9:
NURTURING WELLNESS NATURALLY: EXPLORING SPECIAL TOPICS IN NATURAL REMEDIES

In the intricate journey of health and well-being, Chapter 7 unfolds to delve into special topics within the realm of natural remedies. From managing chronic pain to embracing natural approaches for skin health and understanding the pivotal role of gut health in disease prevention, this chapter explores the harmonious integration of nature's remedies with holistic lifestyle choices.

Managing Chronic Pain: A Symphony of Natural Relief

Chronic pain, an enduring and often challenging condition, casts its shadow over the lives of millions globally. Diverging from the transient discomfort of acute pain, chronic pain persists, its origins often shrouded in ambiguity. Conditions such as arthritis, nerve damage, or the lingering aftermath of past injuries contribute to this relentless ailment. In the pursuit of relief, many turn to natural remedies, seeking alternatives or complements to conventional pain management. Small adjustments in daily habits can wield a profound impact on chronic pain. The rhythmic cadence of low-impact exercises like swimming or yoga emerges as a therapeutic melody, enhancing muscle strength and flexibility, and thereby reducing pain. Adequate sleep and stress management techniques, including meditation and deep-breathing exercises, take center stage, acknowledging their pivotal roles in the symphony of pain relief.

Dietary Approaches: A Nutritional Prelude to Pain Management

Certain foods, with their anti-inflammatory properties, become instrumental in the management of pain. The inclusion of omega-3-rich foods such as fish, flaxseeds, and walnuts, coupled with antioxidants found in berries, nuts, and green leafy vegetables, harmonizes with the body's natural ability to manage pain. Simultaneously, reducing processed foods and sugars, which can exacerbate inflammation, becomes a dietary refrain.

Herbs such as turmeric, ginger, and willow bark, steeped in the annals of history, offer their botanical prowess for pain relief. Laden with compounds that may diminish inflammation and provide respite from pain, these herbal allies beckon individuals on the quest for natural relief. However, the wisdom of consultation with healthcare professionals before incorporating herbal supplements, particularly alongside other medications, is a guiding principle.

The therapeutic trio of acupuncture, massage, and chiropractic care unveils itself as a potent allies in the quest for pain relief. These holistic therapies, akin to melodic movements, alleviate muscle tension, enhance circulation, and awaken the body's innate pain-relieving mechanisms, contributing to the symphony of natural relief. The skin, a sentinel against environmental threats, a regulator of temperature and hydration, becomes the canvas for natural approaches to health. Nurturing the skin from both within and without emerges as a focal point.

Nutrition for Skin Health: A Culinary Overture

A culinary overture unfolds, emphasizing a diet rich in vitamins, minerals, and antioxidants as vital for radiant skin health. Vitamin C-laden oranges and bell peppers, Vitamin E-rich almonds and sunflower seeds, and Omega-3 fatty acids from the embrace of salmon and avocados compose a symphony supporting skin well-being.

The alchemy of natural ingredients, including aloe vera, coconut oil, and shea butter, takes center stage in the realm of skincare. Renowned for their soothing and moisturizing properties, these gentle ingredients replace harsh chemicals and fragrances, offering a serenade to reduce skin irritation and dryness.

A ritual unfolds, involving the fundamental acts of drinking ample water and shielding the skin from the sun. Sunscreens adorned with natural ingredients and protective clothing weave a protective tapestry, preventing sun damage—an endeavor crucial in thwarting the aging process and preserving skin vitality.

Gut Health and Its Symphony in Disease Prevention

The gut, a conductor in the symphony of overall health, orchestrates its influence beyond digestion. Home to the vast community of bacteria known as the gut microbiome, this internal ecosystem holds the key to immunity, mental health, and the prevention of various diseases.

A culinary composition takes center stage, advocating for a diet rich in fiber, fermented foods, and diverse plant-based offerings to foster a flourishing microbiome. Yogurt, kefir, sauerkraut, and fiber-rich fruits and vegetables join the ensemble, nurturing the growth of beneficial bacteria.

Probiotics, the live beneficial bacteria found in select foods and supplements, join hands with prebiotics, fibers that nourish these allies. Together, they create a harmonious gut balance essential for digestion, nutrient absorption, and immune function—an instrumental arrangement in the prevention of diseases ranging from diabetes and obesity to mental health disorders.

Research unveils the pioneering overture that links an unhealthy gut to a spectrum of diseases, encompassing diabetes, obesity, rheumatoid arthritis, and mental health disorders. The maintenance of a healthy gut emerges as an integral component in the tapestry of overall health and disease prevention.

A Holistic Approach: The Symbiosis of Nature's Remedies and Lifestyle

In each of these thematic explorations, the underlying philosophy resonates with a holistic understanding of the body. Natural remedies, embraced in harmony with a healthy lifestyle, paint a vivid canvas of well-being. However, it remains paramount to acknowledge that while these remedies offer substantial benefits, they are not substitutes for professional medical advice or treatment. Consultation with healthcare professionals, especially in the case of severe or chronic conditions, stands as a guiding principle.

As we conclude this chapter, it is essential to broaden our horizons and explore additional dimensions of natural remedies:

- Mind-Body Practices: Techniques such as mindfulness meditation, biofeedback, and progressive muscle relaxation bridge the realms of mental and physical well-being.
- Environmental Well-Being: Embracing eco-friendly practices and fostering a connection with nature contribute to overall well-being and sustainability.
- Holistic Therapies: Practices like Ayurveda, traditional Chinese medicine, and energy healing encompass diverse modalities that consider the interconnectedness of mind, body, and spirit.
- Cognitive Health: Engaging in cognitive exercises, maintaining social connections, and embracing lifelong learning contribute to cognitive well-being and brain health.
- Sleep Hygiene: Prioritizing good sleep habits and creating a conducive sleep environment are integral aspects of overall health and vitality.
- Emotional Wellness: Cultivating emotional resilience, expressing emotions, and seeking support contribute to emotional well-being.
- Detoxification: Incorporating periodic detoxification practices, such as fasting and cleansing diets, supports the body's natural cleansing processes.

In the ever-expanding tapestry of holistic well-being, individuals are invited to explore diverse avenues, each contributing a unique thread to the rich fabric of health and vitality. The journey toward well-being is an ongoing composition, an evolving masterpiece that unfolds with every mindful choice and harmonious integration of nature's remedies within the symphony of life.

HOLISTIC HEALING RECIPES RELATED TO THIS CHAPTER

Harmonizing Chronic Pain Smoothie

Ingredients:
- Pineapple (anti-inflammatory)
- Banana (potassium for muscle health)
- Turmeric (natural pain relief)
- Greek yogurt (protein)

Instructions:
- Blend pineapple, banana, a pinch of turmeric, and Greek yogurt for a smoothie that aims to soothe inflammation and support muscle health.

Calories: Around 250 calories, a tasty and pain-relieving treat.

Skin-Nourishing Salad Ensemble

Ingredients:
- Spinach (rich in vitamins and minerals)
- Oranges (vitamin C boost)
- Almonds (vitamin E)
- Salmon (Omega-3 fatty acids)

Instructions:
- Toss spinach, orange segments, almonds, and grilled salmon.
- Drizzle with a citrus vinaigrette for a skin-nourishing symphony.

Calories: Approximately 350 calories, a vibrant and nutrient-packed salad.

Gut Harmony Smoothie Bowl

Ingredients:
- Yogurt (probiotics)
- Berries (fiber)
- Banana (prebiotics)
- Chia seeds (Omega-3 fatty acids)

Instructions:
- Blend yogurt, berries, banana, and chia seeds.
- Top with granola for a gut-friendly smoothie bowl supporting digestion.

Calories: Around 300 calories, a delicious and gut-nourishing bowl.

Mind-Body Bliss Tea Infusion

Ingredients:
- Chamomile tea (mind relaxation)
- Mint leaves (digestive aid)
- Lemon balm (calming)
- Honey (natural sweetness)

Instructions:
- Brew chamomile tea, add fresh mint leaves, lemon balm, and a teaspoon of honey.
- Sip slowly, embracing the mind-body connection.

Calories: Minimal, around 10-15 calories, a soothing elixir for holistic well-being.

Cognitive Health Granola Bars

Ingredients:
- Oats (fiber)
- Nuts and seeds (brain-boosting Omega 3)
- Dried fruits (antioxidants)
- Dark chocolate (cognitive function)

Instructions:
- Mix oats, nuts, seeds, dried fruits, and dark chocolate chunks.
- Press into bars and bake. These granola bars are a tasty way to support cognitive health.

Calories: Approximately 200 calories per bar, a convenient and brain-boosting snack.
Remember, these recipes are not just about nourishing the body but embodying the holistic principles of well-being. Enjoy these culinary creations as part of your journey toward a healthier, balanced, and harmonious life!

Record your reflections, insights, and observations on the concepts discussed earlier.

Use this space to brainstorm, sketch, or jot down any questions that arise in your mind. Make it a truly personal experience.

CHAPTER 10:
HOLISTIC STRATEGIES IN CANCER CARE: NURTURING HOPE THROUGH NATURAL REMEDIES

Cancer, a complex malady characterized by the unbridled proliferation of abnormal cells, demands a multifaceted approach to treatment and management. While conventional medicine offers surgical interventions, chemotherapy, and radiation therapy, a growing number of individuals and healthcare practitioners are delving into the realm of natural remedies in the pursuit of comprehensive cancer care. These natural approaches seek to fortify the body's inherent healing capabilities, enhance the quality of life, and complement traditional treatments.

Beyond its physical manifestations, cancer touches patients on emotional and spiritual levels. Natural therapies pivot toward treating the entirety of the individual, acknowledging that the impact of cancer extends beyond the physical realm. Ranging from dietary modifications to herbal interventions, these natural practices strive to detoxify the body, bolster the immune system, and provide vital nutrients.

Herbs such as turmeric, celebrated for its active compound curcumin, exhibit promise in laboratory studies for their potential anti-cancer properties. Similarly, green tea, adorned with antioxidants, may confer a protective effect. It is imperative, however, to recognize that while these natural agents display potential, they are not substitutes for conventional cancer treatments but rather allies in supporting overall health.

Integrative Vistas in Cancer Treatment

Integrative oncology emerges as a beacon in the realm of cancer care, blending traditional medical treatments with complementary therapies. This patient-centered approach endeavors to optimize health, enhance quality of life, and improve clinical outcomes throughout the cancer care continuum. A collaborative team, comprising oncologists, dietitians, psychotherapists, and practitioners of alternative therapies, collaborates to craft personalized treatment plans for each patient. Acupuncture, for example, finds application in alleviating chemotherapy-induced nausea and pain. Simultaneously, massage therapy and yoga weave into the fabric of cancer care, diminishing stress and elevating the quality of life for individuals navigating the challenges of cancer.

Nutritional Nourishment for Cancer Warriors

Nutrition emerges as a pivotal player in the symphony of cancer care. A diet rich in fruits, vegetables, whole grains, and lean proteins provides essential nutrients, supports immune function, and aids the body in confronting the side effects of cancer treatments. Berries and leafy greens, brimming with antioxidants, become virtuosos in this nutritional orchestra. Additionally, omega-3 fatty acids, found in fish and flaxseeds, unveil anti-inflammatory properties that prove beneficial for cancer patients.

Individualized dietary approaches, tailored to unique needs and treatment plans, necessitate the guidance of oncology-specialized dietitians. Their expertise ensures a harmonious integration of nutritional support within the overarching strategy of cancer care.

While natural remedies for cancer provide a holistic approach, augmenting traditional treatments, their pursuit demands the guidance of qualified health professionals. The synergy of conventional and natural therapies paints a comprehensive canvas in cancer care, aspiring not merely to treat the disease but to elevate the overall well-being of the patient.

As we draw the curtain on this chapter, it is essential to broaden our perspectives and explore additional dimensions of holistic cancer care:

Physical Fitness Programs: Tailored exercise regimens, designed in collaboration with healthcare professionals, contribute to physical well-being and resilience during cancer treatment.

Environmental Support: Creating a healing environment at home, surrounded by nature and supportive elements, contributes to the overall well-being of cancer patients.

Innovations in Research: Keeping abreast of advancements in cancer research and emerging therapies ensures an informed and empowered approach to treatment decisions.

The journey through cancer is a dynamic composition, and each individual's path is a unique symphony of courage, resilience, and hope. The holistic embrace of natural remedies, entwined with conventional treatments, weaves a tapestry of comprehensive care—a testament to the ongoing pursuit of well-being in the face of adversity.

HOLISTIC HEALING RECIPES RELATED TO THIS CHAPTER

Antioxidant-Packed Smoothie for Cancer Warriors

Ingredients:
* Blueberries (rich in antioxidants)
* Kale (nutrient-dense green)
* Greek yogurt (protein)
* Flaxseeds (omega-3 fatty acids)

Instructions:
* Blend blueberries, kale, Greek yogurt, and a sprinkle of flaxseeds for a nourishing smoothie that supports immune function and provides essential nutrients.

Calories: Approximately 250 calories, a delicious and nutrient-dense drink.

Turmeric-Infused Quinoa Bowl

Ingredients:
- Quinoa (protein and fiber)
- Turmeric-spiced chickpeas (anti-inflammatory)
- Spinach (iron and antioxidants)
- Almonds (vitamin E)

Instructions:
- Cook quinoa and top with turmeric-spiced chickpeas, sautéed spinach, and sliced almonds.
- This bowl is a flavorful and cancer-fighting powerhouse.

Calories: Around 400 calories, a satisfying and nutritious meal.

Omega-3 Salmon Salad

Ingredients:
- Grilled salmon (omega-3 fatty acids)
- Mixed greens (fiber)
- Berries (antioxidants)
- Avocado (healthy fats)

Instructions:
- Assemble mixed greens, grilled salmon, berries, and sliced avocado for a colorful and nutrient-rich salad that supports overall well-being.

Calories: Approximately 350 calories, a light yet fulfilling option.

Detoxifying Green Tea Elixir

Ingredients:
- Green tea (antioxidants)
- Mint leaves (digestive aid)
- Lemon (vitamin C boost)
- Honey (natural sweetness)

Instructions:
- Brew green tea, add fresh mint leaves, a squeeze of lemon, and a teaspoon of honey.
- Sip on this detoxifying elixir for a refreshing and supportive drink.

Calories: Minimal, around 10-15 calories, a soothing beverage for holistic well-being.

Cancer Care Energy Bites

Ingredients:
- Oats (fiber)
- Almond butter (protein)
- Chia seeds (omega-3 fatty acids)
- Dried cranberries (antioxidants)

Instructions:
- Mix oats, almond butter, chia seeds, and dried cranberries.
- Roll into energy bites for a convenient and nutrient-packed snack during cancer care.

Calories: Approximately 150 calories per serving, a wholesome and energizing treat.

Broccoli and Walnut Cancer-Fighting Stir-Fry

Ingredients:
- Broccoli florets (anti-cancer properties)
- Tofu or lean protein of choice
- Walnuts (omega-3 fatty acids)
- Garlic and ginger (anti-inflammatory)

Instructions:
- Stir-fry broccoli, tofu, walnuts, garlic, and ginger in a wok.
- Serve over brown rice or quinoa for a delicious and cancer-fighting stir-fry.

Calories: Around 350 calories, a flavorful and nutritious meal.

Herbal Infused Water for Hydration

Ingredients:
- Cucumber slices (hydration)
- Fresh mint leaves (digestive aid)
- Lemon slices (vitamin C boost)

Instructions:
- Infuse water with cucumber slices, fresh mint leaves, and lemon slices for a refreshing and hydrating herbal elixir.

Calories: Virtually zero, a simple and rejuvenating drink.

Cancer Care Whole Grain Muffins

Ingredients:
- Whole wheat flour (fiber)
- Carrots (beta-carotene)
- Nuts (vitamin E)
- Applesauce (natural sweetness)

Instructions:
- Bake muffins using whole wheat flour, grated carrots, nuts, and applesauce.
- These whole-grain muffins make for a nutritious and easy snack.

Calories: Approximately 150 calories per muffin, a wholesome and convenient option.

Remember, these recipes are designed to support overall well-being during the cancer journey. Always consult with healthcare professionals for personalized advice and treatment plans. Enjoy these wholesome and nourishing creations as part of a comprehensive approach to cancer care.

Record your reflections, insights, and observations on the concepts discussed earlier.

Use this space to brainstorm, sketch, or jot down any questions that arise in your mind. Make it a truly personal experience.

CHAPTER 11:
HARMONY IN HEART HEALTH: EMBRACING NATURE'S SUPPORT FOR CARDIOVASCULAR WELL-BEING

In the symphony of life, the heart takes center stage, orchestrating the vital rhythm that sustains our existence. As heart disease continues to rank among the leading global causes of mortality, a burgeoning interest has emerged in the potential of natural remedies and lifestyle modifications to fortify cardiovascular well-being. Beyond merely preventing or managing heart disease, the focus expands to nurturing the intricate rhythm of this remarkable organ, ensuring it functions optimally.

The heartbeat, a rhythmic dance choreographed by intricate interactions of electrical impulses, muscle function, and blood flow, transcends its surface-level beat. A healthy rhythm signifies the efficient circulation of blood, delivering essential nutrients and oxygen to various organs. Disruption to this rhythm can lead to a spectrum of heart conditions. Fostering a natural and healthy heart rhythm becomes an art, blending elements of good nutrition, regular exercise, stress management, and the avoidance of detrimental habits like smoking. It's about crafting a harmonious lifestyle that reveres and sustains the heart's innate function.

Sculpting Heart Health through Lifestyle Interventions

Diet as a Symphony of Nutrients: A heart-healthy diet, akin to a symphony of nutrients, encompasses fruits, vegetables, whole grains, lean proteins, and heart-friendly fats. Omega-3-rich salmon and antioxidant-packed berries emerge as virtuosos in this nutritional ensemble. The refrain includes minimizing processed foods, salt, and unhealthy fats.

Exercise as the Rhythmic Cadence: The heartbeat of physical activity need not be intense; even the gentle cadence of brisk walking or cycling can fortify the heart. Aiming for at least 150 minutes of moderate aerobic exercise per week becomes a rhythmic melody that strengthens the heart.

Stress Management as a Soothing Melody: The discordant notes of chronic stress can echo negatively in heart health. The soothing melodies of yoga, meditation, and deep breathing exercises become therapeutic harmonies, managing stress levels and fostering cardiovascular well-being.

<u>Sleep as the Restorative Interlude:</u> Amidst the symphony of heart health, adequate and quality sleep emerges as a restorative interlude. Poor sleep patterns, akin to dissonant chords, have been linked to elevated risks of heart disease.

Supplemental Serenades for Cardiovascular Support

In concert with lifestyle changes, certain supplements lend their melodic support:
- <u>Omega-3 Fatty Acids:</u> Extracted from fish oil, these harmonious compounds reduce triglycerides, mildly lower blood pressure, and modulate blood clotting.
- <u>Coenzyme Q10 (CoQ10):</u> A naturally occurring antioxidant, CoQ10 contributes to heart muscle function and blood pressure regulation.
- <u>Magnesium:</u> The essential note for heart rhythm, magnesium orchestrates blood pressure regulation and vitalizes muscle function.
- <u>Garlic:</u> The rhythmic ally known for lowering cholesterol and moderating blood pressure.
- <u>Green Tea Extract:</u> Abounding in antioxidants, this musical extract harmonizes with improved heart health, emphasizing moderation due to its caffeine content.

A Crescendo of Caution and Consultation

While these natural remedies compose a melodious ensemble supporting heart health, they are not substitutes for medical treatment in the context of existing heart conditions. A consultative overture with a healthcare professional before commencing any new supplement, especially for individuals with health concerns or on medication, is imperative.

Caring for the heart transcends a singular note; it entails a symphony of approaches. A balanced diet, regular exercise, stress management, quality sleep, and the potential inclusion of heart-supporting supplements harmonize in a melody that resonates with the heart's natural rhythm. By comprehending and honoring this intrinsic rhythm, we embark on significant strides toward preventing heart disease and nurturing overall health—an ode to the orchestration of a healthy heart.

HOLISTIC HEALING RECIPES RELATED TO THIS CHAPTER

Omega-3 Salmon Salad Serenade

<u>Ingredients:</u>
- Grilled salmon (omega-3 fatty acids)
- Mixed greens (fiber)
- Avocado (heart-friendly fats)
- Berries (antioxidants)

<u>Instructions:</u>
- Assemble mixed greens, grilled salmon, sliced avocado, and a handful of berries.
- Drizzle with olive oil and balsamic vinegar for a heart-healthy salad serenade.

<u>Calories:</u> Approximately 400 calories, a delightful and nutrient-rich ensemble.

Meditative Green Tea Smoothie

<u>Ingredients:</u>
- Green tea (antioxidants)

- Spinach (iron and nutrients)
- Banana (potassium)
- Greek yogurt (protein)

Instructions:
- Brew green tea and let it cool.
- Blend with spinach, banana, and Greek yogurt for a calming and heart-supporting smoothie.

Calories: Around 250 calories, a refreshing and nutritious drink.

Heartfelt Garlic and Herb Quinoa Bowl

Ingredients:
- Quinoa (fiber and protein)
- Grilled chicken or tofu
- Garlic (cholesterol-lowering)
- Fresh herbs (antioxidants)

Instructions:
- Cook quinoa and top with grilled chicken or tofu, sautéed garlic, and a sprinkle of fresh herbs.
- This hearty bowl is a flavorful homage to heart health.

Calories: Approximately 350 calories, a satisfying and wholesome meal.

Magnesium-Packed Dark Chocolate Bliss

Ingredients:
- Dark chocolate (moderation)
- Almonds (magnesium)
- Dried fruits (antioxidants)

Instructions:
- Melt dark chocolate and mix with almonds and dried fruits.
- Allow it to cool and break into pieces for a heart-supporting and indulgent treat.

Calories: Around 200 calories, a delicious and magnesium-rich dessert.

CoQ10 Citrus Smoothie Bowl

Ingredients:
- Oranges (vitamin C)
- Greek yogurt (CoQ10)
- Granola (fiber)
- Chia seeds (omega-3 fatty acids)

Instructions:
- Blend oranges and Greek yogurt.
- Top with granola and chia seeds for a CoQ10-infused smoothie bowl that supports heart muscle function.

Calories: Approximately 300 calories, a vibrant and heart-boosting bowl.

Stress-Busting Berry Yogurt Parfait

Ingredients:
- Greek yogurt (protein)
- Mixed berries (antioxidants)
- Almonds (heart-friendly fats)
- Honey (natural sweetness)

Instructions:
- Layer Greek yogurt with mixed berries, almonds, and a drizzle of honey.
- This parfait not only supports heart health but also contributes to stress management with its soothing combination.

Calories: Around 300 calories, a delightful and nutritious parfait.

Avocado and Tomato Salsa Whole Grain Toast

Ingredients:
- Whole grain bread (fiber)
- Avocado (heart-friendly fats)
- Tomatoes (lycopene)
- Fresh cilantro (antioxidants)

Instructions:
- Toast whole grain bread and top with mashed avocado, diced tomatoes, and fresh cilantro.
- This heart-healthy toast is a flavorful and nourishing choice.

Calories: Approximately 250 calories, a savory and heart-supporting snack.

Mango Turmeric Chia Pudding

Ingredients:
- Chia seeds (omega-3 fatty acids)
- Almond milk (heart-friendly fats)
- Mango (vitamin C)
- Turmeric powder (anti-inflammatory)

Instructions:
- Mix chia seeds with almond milk, diced mango, and a pinch of turmeric powder.
- Allow it to set overnight for a delicious and heart-nurturing chia pudding.

Calories: Around 220 calories, a nutritious and tropical delight.

Enjoy these heart-healthy recipes as part of your journey toward cardiovascular well-being. Remember to consult with healthcare professionals for personalized advice and guidance.

Record your reflections, insights, and observations on the concepts discussed earlier.

Use this space to brainstorm, sketch, or jot down any questions that arise in your mind. Make it a truly personal experience.

CHAPTER 12:
NURTURING WELLNESS: A HOLISTIC APPROACH TO DIABETES MANAGEMENT

Diabetes, marked by elevated blood sugar levels, unfolds as a complex journey demanding not just numerical management but a profound shift in lifestyle. Fortunately, nature unfolds an array of tools to fortify this battle, delving into the realms of balancing blood sugar naturally, integrating supplements, and embracing transformative lifestyle changes as potent strategies in the management of diabetes.

At the heart of diabetes management lies the art of blood sugar control—a quest to maintain a harmonious glucose level, steering clear of spikes and drops. The journey commences with deciphering the glycemic index (GI) of foods, unveiling the tempo at which they influence blood sugar levels. Embracing low GI foods, such as fiber-rich whole grains, legumes, and abundant vegetables, forms the melodic foundation. Beyond impeding rapid glucose absorption, these foods satiate, curbing the temptation to indulge in sugary treats.

In the symphony of diabetes management, vigilant monitoring emerges as the keynote of insight. Regularly tracking blood sugar levels becomes a virtuoso practice, unraveling the intricate interplay between different foods and activities and their impact on the body. This profound understanding paves the way for informed choices, both in dietary selections and lifestyle pursuits.

Supplemental Harmonies from Nature's Apothecary

Nature's apothecary generously offers supplements harmonizing with blood sugar control:

Cinnamon: Beyond a Culinary Spice: Elevating cinnamon beyond its culinary role, studies illuminate its positive influence on blood sugar levels. Enhancing insulin sensitivity, cinnamon empowers the body's cells to more efficiently utilize available sugar.

Bitter Melon: A Vegetable Symphony: Despite its acquired taste, bitter melon takes center stage for its glucose-lowering prowess. Laden with compounds resembling insulin, bitter melon plays a symphony in lowering blood sugar levels.

Magnesium: The Elemental Cadence: Recognizing the commonality of low magnesium levels in diabetes, supplementation emerges as a cadence of elemental support. Improving insulin sensitivity, magnesium serves as a preventive measure against diabetes-related complications.

Omega-3 Fatty Acids: The Overture of Heart and Sugar Health: Resonating not only with cardiovascular well-being but also with blood sugar regulation, omega-3 fatty acids, sourced from fish oil and flaxseeds, compose an overture of holistic health.

While these supplements weave harmonies in support of blood sugar control, they are not substitutes but complementary notes to standard diabetes treatments. A consultation with healthcare providers before introducing any new supplement is a precautionary crescendo, particularly for individuals with existing health concerns or on medications.

Lifestyle Transformations: The Crescendo of Power

Lifestyle modifications, akin to a crescendo of power, emerge as the most potent tools in the diabetes management ensemble. Key changes unfold as transformative melodies:

- Exercise: A Dance of Glucose Utilization: From cardio to strength training and flexibility exercises, the dance of regular physical activity consumes glucose for energy and muscle building, lowering blood sugar levels.
- Weight Management: A Subtle Impact: Even a modest weight loss, if overweight, orchestrates a profound impact on blood sugar control.
- Stress Management: Harmonizing Cortisol and Glucose: As stress disrupts blood sugar levels, the harmonies of yoga, meditation, and deep breathing exercises offer soothing notes.
- Sleep Quality: The Restorative Serenade: In the nocturnal serenade, 7-8 hours of quality sleep harmonize with blood sugar levels and insulin sensitivity.

In the closing cadence, managing diabetes naturally unveils as a symphony—a comprehensive composition intertwining diet, supplements, and lifestyle changes. It's about striking a balance, attuning to the body's rhythms, and orchestrating adjustments tailored to individual needs. Armed with the right strategies, diabetes transforms from a challenge to a manageable journey, paving the way for a life rich in health and fulfillment.

HOLISTIC HEALING RECIPES RELATED TO THIS CHAPTER

Quinoa and Vegetable Stir-Fry

Ingredients:
- Quinoa (low GI)
- Colorful bell peppers (fiber)
- Broccoli and carrots (vitamins)
- Tofu or lean chicken (protein)

Instructions:
- Stir-fry quinoa with a mix of colorful vegetables and your choice of protein.
- Season with a light soy sauce or a dash of olive oil. This dish is a nutrient-packed and low-GI option for a satisfying meal.

Calories: Approximately 350 calories, a wholesome and diabetes-friendly stir-fry.

Chia Seed Pudding with Berries

Ingredients:
- Chia seeds (fiber)
- Almond milk (unsweetened)
- Mixed berries (antioxidants)
- Nuts or seeds (optional, for added crunch)

Instructions:
- Mix chia seeds with almond milk and let it sit in the fridge overnight.
- Top with mixed berries and a sprinkle of nuts or seeds. This chia seed pudding is a delicious and low-GI dessert or breakfast option.

Calories: Around 250 calories, a tasty and blood sugar-friendly treat.

Vegetarian Lentil Soup

Ingredients:
- Lentils (fiber and protein)
- Tomatoes and carrots (vitamins)
- Spinach or kale (iron)
- Vegetable broth (low sodium)

Instructions:
- Simmer lentils with tomatoes, carrots, spinach or kale, and low-sodium vegetable broth.
- Season with herbs and spices. This hearty lentil soup is a comforting and diabetes-conscious choice.

Calories: Approximately 300 calories, a nutritious and filling soup.

Baked Salmon with Lemon and Herbs

Ingredients:
- Salmon fillets (omega-3 fatty acids)
- Fresh lemon
- Fresh herbs (such as dill or parsley)
- Olive oil (heart-friendly fats)

Instructions:
- Marinate salmon with lemon, fresh herbs, and a drizzle of olive oil.
- Bake until the salmon is cooked through. This flavorful and omega-3-rich dish is a great addition to a diabetes-friendly menu.

Calories: Around 400 calories, a delicious and heart-healthy choice.

Mango and Avocado Salad

Ingredients:
- Mixed greens (fiber)
- Mango (vitamin C)
- Avocado (heart-friendly fats)

- Walnuts or almonds (optional, for added crunch)

Instructions:
- Toss mixed greens with diced mango, sliced avocado, and nuts if desired.
- Dress with a light vinaigrette. This refreshing salad is a vibrant and nutrient-packed addition to your diabetes-conscious meals.

Calories: Approximately 300 calories, a colorful and diabetes-friendly salad.

Whole Grain Vegetable Wrap

Ingredients:
- Whole grain tortilla (low GI)
- Grilled chicken or tofu (protein)
- Sautéed colorful bell peppers and zucchini (fiber)
- Hummus or Greek yogurt dressing

Instructions:
- Fill a whole grain tortilla with grilled chicken or tofu, sautéed vegetables, and a dollop of hummus or a drizzle of Greek yogurt dressing.
- Roll it up for a delicious and diabetes-friendly wrap.

Calories: Around 350 calories, a satisfying and balanced meal.

Cauliflower Fried Rice

Ingredients:
- Cauliflower rice (low-carb)
- Shrimp or tofu (protein)
- Mixed vegetables (such as peas, carrots, and bell peppers)
- Egg (optional)
- Low-sodium soy sauce

Instructions:
- Sauté cauliflower rice with shrimp or tofu, mixed vegetables, and scrambled egg if desired.
- Season with low-sodium soy sauce for a tasty and low-carb alternative to traditional fried rice.

Calories: Approximately 300 calories, a flavorful and diabetes-conscious option.

These recipes, combined with the principles of low GI foods and lifestyle modifications, contribute to a comprehensive approach to diabetes management. As always, consult with healthcare professionals for personalized advice and guidance.

Record your reflections, insights, and observations on the concepts discussed earlier.

Use this space to brainstorm, sketch, or jot down any questions that arise in your mind. Make it a truly personal experience.

CHAPTER 13:
PROACTIVE HEALTH GUARDIANSHIP: A SYMPHONY OF PREVENTION

In the realm of health management, the timeless wisdom of "prevention is better than cure" resonates with unparalleled relevance. In a world grappling with the prevalence of chronic diseases like cancer, heart disease, and diabetes, the imperative to take proactive measures to avert these conditions emerges as paramount. This chapter embarks on an exploration of potent prevention strategies, intricately woven to prioritize health and well-being long before the shadows of disease appear. We will unravel the art of preemptive health care, underscore the significance of early detection, and delve into natural remedies poised to fortify the immune system.

The inaugural defense line in the saga of disease prevention unfolds through lifestyle choices. Daily habits become the architects of your health destiny, wielding profound influence over the likelihood of various health conditions. Here's the blueprint for crafting a lifestyle conducive to disease prevention:

Nutrition: A Symphony of Nourishment: Opt for a symphony of nutrition, where fruits, vegetables, whole grains, and lean proteins take center stage. Laden with essential nutrients, this orchestration supports overall health, erecting a formidable barrier against diseases.

Physical Activity: The Dance of Vitality: Key to disease prevention is the dance of regular exercise. It need not be a strenuous performance; even moderate activities like brisk walking or cycling compose substantial movements on the health stage.

Stress Management: The Serenade of Equanimity: Chronic stress, a silent assailant, weakens the body's defenses. The serenade of stress management techniques—be it through deep breathing—harmonizes the mind, fostering resilience against illnesses.

Adequate Sleep: The Nocturne of Restoration: Quality sleep emerges as the nocturne of restoration, facilitating the repair and rejuvenation of the body. Aiming for 7-8 hours of uninterrupted sleep each night sets the stage for optimal well-being.

<u>Avoiding Harmful Substances:</u> The Overture of Abstinence: In the overture of disease prevention, and bidding farewell to smoking play pivotal roles. These abstentions resonate as powerful notes safeguarding against the onslaught of illnesses.

Early Detection and the Herbal Melodies of Nature

A crescendo in the pursuit of prevention is the timely detection of health issues. Regular health check-ups and screenings, especially with a family history of certain diseases, form the backbone of this vigilance. Accompanying these early detection endeavors are the herbal melodies of nature:

<u>Herbal Supplements:</u> Nature's Elixirs: Herbs like turmeric, ginger, and garlic step forward with anti-inflammatory and antioxidant properties, serving as elixirs in the symphony of natural remedies.

<u>Functional Foods:</u> Culinary Acolytes of Health: The culinary acolytes—blueberries, nuts, and green tea—enrich the symphony with their health-promoting properties, complementing early detection efforts.

<u>Mind-Body Practices:</u> The Ballet of Harmony: Techniques like Tai Chi and Qi Gong orchestrate a ballet of mental and physical well-being, enhancing early detection through heightened body awareness.

Nurturing the Bastion: A Robust Immune System

At the heart of disease prevention stands a robust immune system, an impregnable bastion against illnesses. The fortification unfolds through:
- <u>Nutrient-Rich Diet:</u> The Feast of Vitality: A feast rich in vitamins and minerals, particularly vitamin C, vitamin D, zinc, and selenium, is the sustenance for a robust immune system.
- <u>Regular Exercise:</u> The Anthem of Vitality: Beyond physical fitness, regular exercise becomes the anthem of vitality, elevating immune response to the crescendo of optimal health.
- <u>Adequate Sleep and Hydration:</u> The Hydration Sonata: The hydration sonata, complemented by adequate sleep, conducts the symphony of optimal immune function.
- <u>Probiotics:</u> Guardians of Gut Health: Probiotics, the guardians of gut health, take center stage in the symphony of immune function, reinforcing the link between a healthy gut and a resilient immune system.
- <u>Reducing Stress:</u> The Lullaby of Equilibrium: As chronic stress weakens the immune system, the lullaby of stress management emerges as the key to sustaining good health.

Prevention strategies unfold as an art—a symphony of health where every note, every lifestyle choice, every moment of vigilance contributes to the masterpiece. By embracing healthy lifestyle choices, maintaining vigilance through early detection, and nurturing the immune system, the foundation is laid for a life rich in health and free from the shackles of disease. Each small step in this journey becomes a significant note in the opus of overall well-being.

HOLISTIC HEALING RECIPES RELATED TO THIS CHAPTER

Vitality Smoothie Bowl

<u>Ingredients:</u>
- Greek yogurt (protein)
- Mixed berries (antioxidants)

- Spinach (vitamins and minerals)
- Chia seeds (omega-3 fatty acids)

Instructions:
- Blend Greek yogurt with mixed berries and a handful of spinach.
- Pour the smoothie into a bowl and top it with chia seeds for an extra boost of omega-3 fatty acids.
- This vitality smoothie bowl is rich in nutrients to support overall health.

Calories: Around 300 calories, a vibrant and nutrient-packed breakfast.

Immune-Boosting Salad

Ingredients:
- Kale or mixed greens (fiber and vitamins)
- Quinoa (protein and fiber)
- Cherry tomatoes (vitamin C)
- Avocado (healthy fats)
- Walnuts (omega-3 fatty acids)

Instructions:
- Toss kale or mixed greens with cooked quinoa, cherry tomatoes, sliced avocado, and walnuts.
- Drizzle with a light vinaigrette for a delicious and immune-boosting salad.

Calories: Approximately 350 calories, a nutrient-dense lunch or dinner option.

Hydration Infusion

Ingredients:
- Cucumber slices
- Lemon or lime slices
- Fresh mint leaves
- Ginger slices

Instructions:
- Combine cucumber slices, lemon or lime slices, fresh mint leaves, and ginger slices in a pitcher of water.
- Let it infuse for a few hours in the refrigerator.
- This hydration infusion is a refreshing and low-calorie way to stay hydrated.

Calories: Virtually calorie-free, a hydrating and flavorful beverage.

Turmeric-Ginger Tea

Ingredients:
- Turmeric powder
- Fresh ginger slices
- Honey (optional)

Instructions:
- Brew a cup of hot water and add turmeric powder and fresh ginger slices.
- Allow it to steep for a few minutes.

- Add honey for sweetness if desired. Turmeric and ginger have anti-inflammatory properties, making this tea a soothing and healthful beverage.

Calories: Minimal calories, a warm and comforting drink.

Probiotic-Packed Yogurt Parfait

Ingredients:
- Greek yogurt (probiotics)
- Berries (antioxidants)
- Almond granola (fiber and healthy fats)

Instructions:
- Layer Greek yogurt with fresh berries and almond granola in a glass or bowl.
- This probiotic-packed parfait is not only delicious but also supports gut health.

Calories: Around 250 calories, a satisfying and gut-friendly snack.

Antioxidant-Packed Breakfast Smoothie

Ingredients:
- Blueberries (antioxidants)
- Banana (vitamins and minerals)
- Kale (fiber and nutrients)
- Flaxseeds (omega-3 fatty acids)

Instructions:
- Blend blueberries, banana, kale, and a sprinkle of flaxseeds with your choice of milk or yogurt.
- This smoothie is bursting with antioxidants, vitamins, and omega-3 fatty acids to kickstart your day.

Calories: Around 250 calories, a refreshing and nutrient-dense morning option.

Mediterranean Quinoa Salad

Ingredients:
- Quinoa (protein and fiber)
- Cherry tomatoes (vitamin C)
- Cucumber (hydration)
- Kalamata olives (healthy fats)
- Feta cheese (calcium and probiotics)

Instructions:
- Cook quinoa and let it cool.
- Mix it with cherry tomatoes, cucumber, Kalamata olives, and crumbled feta cheese.
- Drizzle with olive oil and a squeeze of lemon for a Mediterranean-inspired, nutrient-rich salad.

Calories: Approximately 300 calories, a satisfying and colorful lunch.

These recipes align with the prevention strategies discussed in the chapter, emphasizing nutrient-rich ingredients, antioxidants, and immune-boosting elements. As always, tailor these recipes to individual preferences and consult healthcare professionals for personalized advice.

Record your reflections, insights, and observations on the concepts discussed earlier.

Use this space to brainstorm, sketch, or jot down any questions that arise in your mind. Make it a truly personal experience.

CHAPTER 14:
CRAFTING YOUR PERSONALIZED PATH TO NATURAL WELLNESS

Embarking on the journey of creating your own natural remedy plan is a profound exploration, a harmonious blend of ancient wisdom and modern health insights. This chapter invites you to seize the reins of your well-being narrative, to delve into the realms of personalized health, and to unearth natural ways to fortify the innate healing processes of your body.

Assessing Your Health Mosaic

The inaugural step in this odyssey is akin to taking a panoramic snapshot of your current health landscape. Let's dive into the multi-faceted aspects:

Medical Tapestry: Unraveling Your History: Conduct a meticulous review of your medical history, unveiling the tapestry of past and present medical conditions, surgeries, and treatments. This historical perspective lays the groundwork for understanding your body's unique story.

Lifestyle Kaleidoscope: Illuminating Daily Habits: Illuminate the kaleidoscope of your daily habits, from the culinary choices that grace your plate to the cadence of your exercise routine. Observe the patterns of sleep, scrutinize stress levels, and sketch the contours of your lifestyle canvas.

Symphonic Self-Check: Tuning Into Your Body: Conduct a symphonic self-check, tuning into the subtle notes of your body. Note down even the seemingly minor symptoms that play a part in your daily narrative. This attentive listening forms the melody of your health status.

Professional Prelude: Insight Through Assessment: If feasible, embark on a professional health assessment, a prelude orchestrated through blood tests and expert evaluations. This symphony of insights provides a detailed score, enriching your understanding of your health orchestra.

The essence lies in gathering a symphony of information, creating a resonance that becomes the foundation upon which your natural remedy plan will be orchestrated.

Setting Sail with Personal Health Constellations

Now, let's navigate the celestial expanse of health goals. This isn't about reaching for unreachable stars but about sculpting realistic constellations, and guiding your journey:

Constellations of Vitality: Realistic and Attainable: Identify diverse health goals, ranging from enhancing energy levels to mitigating specific symptoms. These constellations could involve achieving dietary equilibrium, fortifying mental well-being, or sculpting physical strength.

SMART Navigation: Charting the Course: Navigate through the cosmos of health goals with the SMART compass—making them Specific, Measurable, Achievable, Relevant, and Time-bound. Transform abstract aspirations into tangible endeavors. For instance, shift from "I want to be healthier" to "I aim to walk 30 minutes daily for the next three months to improve cardiovascular health."

Crafting the Symphony: Your Personal Remedy Plan

The crescendo of action comes to life as you craft your personalized remedy plan. Translate assessments and goals into a tangible composition:

Dietary Harmonies: Composing a Nourishing Score: Harmonize your diet based on health assessments. Compose a score that resonates with your body's needs—perhaps integrating anti-inflammatory foods or moderating sugar intake.

Herbal Sonnets: The Elixir of Nature: Conduct a poetic exploration of herbs that could be instrumental in your health journey. Remember, consultation with a healthcare provider is a crucial refrain before introducing any new supplement, especially if melodies of existing conditions or medications play in your health composition.

Lifestyle Ballet: Choreographing Well-being: Choreograph lifestyle changes that dance in tandem with your goals. This could involve a new exercise routine pirouetting into your life, improvements in sleep choreography, or the calming pirouettes of stress-reduction techniques.

Progress Sonata: Monitoring the Symphony: Compose a progress sonata, a harmonious melody tracking your journey. Whether through the written notes of a health journal, the digital rhythm of an app, or the collaborative symphony with a health professional, monitoring becomes the rhythm that guides your cadence.

Adaptation Symphony: Tuning Into Feedback: Prepare for the adaptation symphony, where your body becomes the maestro. Listen to the feedback, and with the grace of an artist, adjust your plan accordingly. Flexibility and adaptation become the key notes in this evolving melody.

In crafting this plan, remember, this journey is yours and yours alone. What resonates with one soul may not harmonize with another, and that's the beauty of the symphony of health. Always engage the expertise of healthcare professionals when orchestrating significant changes in your health composition. With the virtuosity of patience, the persistence of practice, and a touch of experimentation, you are poised to compose a natural remedy plan, an opus that resonates with your unique journey toward holistic health.

HOLISTIC HEALING RECIPES RELATED TO THIS CHAPTER

Herbal Symphony Recipe: Immune-Boosting Tea

Ingredients:
- Echinacea (immune support)
- Elderberry (antioxidant-rich)
- Ginger (anti-inflammatory)
- Lemon (vitamin C)

Instructions:
- Steep echinacea, elderberry, and ginger in hot water.
- Squeeze fresh lemon juice into the mixture.
- Strain and enjoy this immune-boosting tea daily.

Calories: Virtually calorie-free, this herbal tea provides a soothing and health-enhancing beverage option.

Nutrient-Packed Meal: Quinoa and Vegetable Bowl

Ingredients:
- Quinoa (fiber and protein)
- Spinach (iron and vitamins)
- Bell peppers (vitamin C)
- Chickpeas (protein and fiber)
- Avocado (healthy fats)

Instructions:
- Cook quinoa and arrange it as a base in a bowl.
- Top with sautéed spinach, bell peppers, and chickpeas.
- Garnish with avocado slices for a nourishing and balanced meal.

Calories: Approximately 400 calories, a wholesome and nutrient-dense bowl.

Adaptogenic Elixir: Ashwagandha Infused Smoothie

Ingredients:
- Ashwagandha powder (adaptogen)
- Banana (potassium and energy)
- Almond milk
- Mixed berries (antioxidants)

Instructions:
- Blend ashwagandha powder, banana, and mixed berries with almond milk.
- This adaptogenic smoothie supports stress management and provides a nutrient boost.

Calories: Around 300 calories, a delicious and stress-relieving smoothie.

Sleep-Inducing Ritual: Lavender-Infused Bedtime Tea

Ingredients:

- Chamomile tea bags (calming)
- Lavender buds (stress relief)
- Honey (optional, for sweetness)

Instructions:
- Steep chamomile tea bags and lavender buds in hot water.
- Add honey if desired.
- Enjoy this calming bedtime tea for a restful night's sleep.

Calories: Virtually calorie-free, promoting relaxation and aiding in quality sleep.

Immune-Boosting Citrus Salad

Ingredients:
- Mixed citrus fruits (vitamin C)
- Kale (nutrient-rich greens)
- Walnuts (omega-3 fatty acids)
- Feta cheese (calcium and protein)
- Olive oil and balsamic vinegar dressing

Instructions:
- Toss together mixed citrus fruits, chopped kale, and walnuts.
- Crumble feta cheese on top.
- Drizzle with olive oil and balsamic vinegar dressing.
- Enjoy this refreshing and immune-boosting citrus salad.

Calories: Approximately 300 calories, a zesty and nutritious salad.

Mood-Boosting Dark Chocolate Energy Bites

Ingredients:
- Rolled oats (fiber and energy)
- Dark chocolate (antioxidants)
- Almond butter (healthy fats and protein)
- Chia seeds (omega-3)
- Honey (natural sweetener)

Instructions:
- Mix rolled oats, melted dark chocolate, almond butter, chia seeds, and honey.
- Form into bite-sized balls and refrigerate.
- These energy bites serve as a mood-boosting and satisfying snack.

Calories: Around 150 calories per serving, a guilt-free indulgence.

These additions provide practical elements to the chapter, offering readers tangible examples of how to incorporate natural remedies into their daily lives. Each suggestion aligns with the overall theme of crafting a personalized and holistic health plan.

Record your reflections, insights, and observations on the concepts discussed earlier.

Use this space to brainstorm, sketch, or jot down any questions that arise in your mind. Make it a truly personal experience.

CHAPTER 15:
RECIPES FOR SPECIFIC HEALTH CONDITION

HEALTHY DIABETES-FRIENDLY RECIPES

One-Pot White Bean, Spinach & Sun-Dried Tomato Orzo with Lemon & Feta

Whip up a delightful one-pot pasta featuring white beans, spinach, and sun-dried tomatoes. It's a burst of flavors that not only tantalizes your taste buds but also makes cleanup a breeze. Elevate the dish by toasting the orzo beforehand, enhancing its richness. Swap out spinach for robust greens like chopped kale or Swiss chard, though be mindful of their cooking time—add them to the pan during the final 5 minutes.

Active Time: 25 mins
Total Time: 40 mins
Servings: 6

Ingredients:
- 1 1/2 tablespoons extra-virgin olive oil
- 1 cup chopped red onion
- 6 cloves garlic, minced
- 1 cup whole-wheat orzo
- 1 cup chopped sun-dried tomatoes
- 2 3/4 cups vegetable broth
- 2 (15-ounce) cans no-salt-added cannellini beans, rinsed
- 1 teaspoon lemon zest
- 3 tablespoons lemon juice
- 3/4 teaspoon salt
- 1/2 teaspoon dried oregano
- 1 (5-ounce) package baby spinach
- 1/4 cup crumbled feta cheese

- 1/2 cup chopped fresh basil
- 1/4 cup toasted pine nuts

Instructions:

1. Start by heating oil in a spacious nonstick skillet over medium heat. Sauté onions until they become aromatic and translucent, which should take around 8 minutes. Introduce garlic to the mix and continue stirring until its fragrance fills the air, about 1 minute.

2. Now, incorporate orzo and sun-dried tomatoes, stirring consistently until the orzo achieves a toasty perfection, approximately 1 minute. Pour in broth, beans, lemon juice, salt, and oregano, then bring the concoction to a lively boil over medium-high heat. Once bubbling, reduce the heat to medium-low, cover the skillet, and let it simmer until the orzo reaches that ideal al dente texture, roughly 15 minutes.

3. In the final stretch, add spinach to the mix. Allow it to wilt by cooking uncovered and stirring occasionally, taking only about 1 minute. When everything is beautifully blended, remove the skillet from heat and generously crown your creation with feta, basil, pine nuts, and a sprinkle of lemon zest.

Nutrition Information: Serving Size: 1 cup
Calories 496, Fat 23g, Saturated Fat 1g, Cholesterol 4mg, Carbohydrates 60g, Total Sugars 14g, Added Sugars 0g, Protein 17g, Fiber 11g, Sodium 480mg, Potassium 895mg

Quick & Spicy Brussels Sprouts with Lemon

Discover the magic of a "reverse sear" with this speedy vegetable side dish! Steam the veggies first to ensure tenderness, then give them a swift sear for that perfect touch without the fear of burning. The added bonus? The microwave takes away the need for boiling water and a steamer basket, making it quick, easy, and all-in-one!

Active Time: 15 mins
Total Time: 15 mins
Servings: 4

Ingredients:
- 1 pound Brussels sprouts, trimmed and halved lengthwise (quartered, if large)
- 1 tablespoon water
- 2 tablespoons extra-virgin olive oil
- 1/2 teaspoon salt
- 1/4 teaspoon crushed red pepper
- 1/2 teaspoon lemon zest
- 1 teaspoon lemon juice

Instructions:

1. Begin by placing Brussels sprouts and water in a microwave-safe bowl. Cover and microwave on High for approximately 3 minutes, ensuring they turn a vibrant green while maintaining a crisp texture. Drain the sprouts carefully and pat them dry with a paper towel.

2. Next, heat oil in a spacious nonstick skillet over medium-high heat until it shimmers. Add the drained sprouts, along with salt and crushed red pepper, tossing them to coat in the flavorful oil. Arrange the sprouts with the cut sides down, allowing them to cook undisturbed until browned for 2 to 3 minutes. Stir and continue cooking, occasionally stirring, until they are both tender when pierced with a fork and evenly browned, taking about 3 to 4 minutes.

3. Finally, transfer the beautifully cooked sprouts to a platter. Drizzle them with lemon juice and sprinkle some lemon zest for that extra burst of freshness.

Nutrition Facts (per serving): 109 Calories / 7g Fat / 10g Carbs / 4g Protein

Lemony Lentil & Cauliflower Cup Soup Is an Easy High-Fiber Lunch Idea

Infused with zesty lemon goodness, this soup achieves a delightful blend of fiber and nutty flavor courtesy of lentils and bulgur. Bulgur not only adds a hearty touch but also brings a pleasant chewiness to the texture. Feel free to substitute it with alternatives like brown rice or quinoa for a different twist. The broth receives a subtle kick from harissa paste, imparting a gentle heat. If you're not keen on carrying vegetable broth or lack a microwave, opt for reduced-sodium bouillon and simply mix it with hot water for a convenient solution.

Active Time: 20 mins
Total Time: 30 mins
Servings: 3 servings

Ingredients:
- 1 tablespoon extra-virgin olive oil
- 2 cups chopped cauliflower florets
- 3/4 cup chopped yellow onion
- 2 teaspoons minced garlic
- 1/4 teaspoon salt
- 2 tablespoons water
- 1 cup cooked bulgur
- 1 cup cooked lentils
- 3 tablespoons chopped fresh cilantro
- 2 tablespoons mild harissa paste
- 1 tablespoon lemon juice
- 3 slices lemon
- 3 cups reduced-sodium vegetable broth

Instructions:
1. In a spacious nonstick skillet over medium heat, heat oil. Add cauliflower and onion, stirring occasionally, until they take on a light brown hue and start to soften, around 10 minutes. Stir in garlic and salt, allowing the aroma to infuse for about 1 minute. Pour in water, cover, and let it cook undisturbed until the cauliflower reaches a tender state, approximately 5 minutes. Remove from heat.

2. Portion out bulgur and lentils into 3 (1-pint) canning jars or airtight containers suitable for the microwave. Layer each with 1/2 cup of the cauliflower mixture, 1 tablespoon of cilantro, 2 teaspoons of harissa, 1 teaspoon of lemon juice, and a lemon slice. Cover and refrigerate for up to 3 days.

3. When ready to enjoy a jar of soup, add 1 cup of broth to the jar. Microwave, uncovered, on High in 1-minute intervals, stirring between each, until the soup is piping hot, taking approximately 2 to 3 minutes. Allow it to cool for 5 minutes before savoring the flavors.

To make ahead: Prepare through Step 2. Refrigerate covered jars for up to 3 days.
Equipment: 3 (1-pint) canning jars or microwaveable airtight containers.
Nutrition Information: Serving Size: 1 1/2 cups.

Calories 221, Fat 5g, Saturated Fat 1g, Cholesterol 0mg, Carbohydrates 35g, Total Sugars 7g, Added Sugars 0g, Protein 10g, Fiber 10g, Sodium 415mg, Potassium 575mg

Easy Green Tortellini Soup to Balance Blood Sugar (Make Ahead!)

Prepare the foundation of this vibrant tortellini soup in advance, storing it in separate containers for a convenient, on-the-go lunch option. To prevent the tortellini from becoming soggy, create a protective layer by placing spinach on top of the pesto. When the time comes to indulge, add the broth and heat it up in the microwave. Not only is this recipe low in saturated fat, crucial for individuals with specific health concerns like diabetes, but it also boasts a healthy dose of carbohydrates to maintain steady blood sugar levels, ensuring a consistent and sustained energy supply.

Active Time: 15 mins
Total Time: 20 mins
Servings: 4 servings

Ingredients:
- 4 tablespoons basil pesto
- 2 tablespoons lemon juice
- 2 cups refrigerated spinach-and-cheese tortellini
- 1 cup packed chopped spinach
- 1 cup frozen green peas
- 1/2 cup scallions
- 3 cups unsalted vegetable broth, divided

Instructions:
1. Distribute pesto and lemon juice equally among 4 (1-pint) canning jars or airtight containers suitable for the microwave; mix well. Create layers in each jar with 1/2 cup of tortellini, 1/4 cup of spinach, 1/4 cup of peas, and 2 tablespoons of scallions. Cover and refrigerate for up to 3 days.

2. When ready to enjoy a jar of soup, add 3/4 cup of broth to the jar. Microwave, uncovered, on High in 1-minute intervals, stirring between each, until the soup reaches steaming hotness and the tortellini achieves tenderness, typically taking 4 to 5 minutes in total. Allow it to cool for 5 minutes before serving.

To make ahead: Prepare through Step 1. Refrigerate covered jars for up to 3 days.
Equipment: 4 (1-pint) canning jars or microwaveable airtight containers.

The Best Veggie Enchiladas You'll Ever Make

Loaded with a medley of sweet corn, onions, peppers, zucchini, and beans, these vegetable enchiladas are a flavor-packed delight. To streamline the preparation, they're generously coated with store-bought enchilada sauce. Whether you opt for the earthy notes of red enchilada sauce or the vibrant alternative of green enchilada sauce, the choice is yours. For a unique twist, consider swapping yellow squash for zucchini and introducing a poblano pepper instead of the bell pepper. Customize to your taste!

Active Time: 40 mins
Total Time: 1 hr 5 mins
Servings: 4

Are Corn and Black Beans Beneficial for Your Health?

Despite their reputation for causing some discomfort, beans, including black beans, offer a nutritional powerhouse. Packed with essential vitamins, minerals, antioxidants, and fiber, beans bring a multitude of health benefits. Regular consumption of black beans can enhance gut health, bolster the immune system, and reduce inflammation—potentially lowering the risk of chronic diseases like heart disease and cancer. The fiber content aids in reducing cholesterol, while the potassium in beans helps maintain healthy blood pressure levels. Additionally, incorporating beans into your diet may contribute to stabilized blood sugar and a decreased risk of type 2 diabetes.

Dispelling Corn's Nutrition Myth: Contrary to its undeserved reputation, corn is far from nutritionally empty. This low-fat food contains a mix of saturated, monounsaturated, and polyunsaturated fats. Nearly half of the fat content is polyunsaturated, and both mono- and polyunsaturated fats are heart-healthy. Corn is also rich in fiber and resistant starch, a slowly digesting carbohydrate that promotes a lasting feeling of fullness. Furthermore, corn boasts antioxidants, particularly lutein and zeaxanthin, which play a role in protecting vision.

Unraveling the Health Aspects of Red Enchilada Sauce: Red enchilada sauce is crafted from nutrient-dense ingredients, typically featuring tomato puree, vinegar, and spices. Tomatoes, with their vibrant color, are rich in antioxidants, serving as an excellent source of vitamin C and a good source of vitamin K and potassium. These nutrients collectively support heart health, helping to lower blood pressure and reduce the risk of stroke. The spices and herbs in red enchilada sauce contribute to inflammation reduction. However, it's important to be mindful of sodium content; opt for sauces with less than 300 mg per serving.

Exploring the Nutritional Value of Cheese: Cheese, recognized for its protein and calcium content, also contains probiotics—beneficial bacteria that enhance gut health and overall well-being. While cheese tends to be high in saturated fat, some evidence suggests that the type of saturated fat in cheese may not be harmful and might even offer heart-related benefits.

Insights from the Test Kitchen:

Choosing Enchilada Filling Vegetables: Our recipe features orange bell pepper, red onion, zucchini, corn, and black beans, but feel free to customize. Substitute yellow squash for zucchini or opt for a poblano pepper to add some heat. Consider using no-salt-added pinto beans for a creamy, earthy flavor alternative in the enchiladas.

Selecting the Right Tortillas: Corn tortillas are ideal for this recipe, whether store-bought or homemade. While flour tortillas can be used, note that it will alter the nutritional profile of the dish.

Addressing Common Questions:

Assembling Veggie Enchiladas: To prevent the veggie enchiladas from falling apart during assembly, place the filled tortillas seam-side down in the prepared baking dish.

Ingredients:
- 1 tablespoon extra-virgin olive oil
- 1 small orange bell pepper, chopped
- 1 small red onion, chopped
- 1 small zucchini, halved lengthwise and sliced 1/4-inch thick
- 1 cup corn, fresh or thawed frozen

- 1 teaspoon chili powder
- 1/4 teaspoon salt
- 1 (15 ounce) can no-salt-added black beans, rinsed
- 2 tablespoons chopped fresh cilantro, plus more for garnish
- 8 (6-inch) yellow corn tortillas, warmed
- 1 (10-ounce) can red enchilada sauce (see Tip)
- 3/4 cup shredded Monterey Jack cheese

Instructions:
1. Begin by preheating the oven to 425°F and lightly coating a 7-by-11-inch baking dish with cooking spray. In a large skillet over medium-high heat, heat oil. Add bell pepper and onion, stirring occasionally, until softened for approximately 5 minutes. Introduce zucchini, corn, chili powder, and salt; continue to cook, stirring occasionally, until the zucchini and corn reach a tender-crisp state, taking about 5 minutes. Remove from heat and stir in beans and cilantro. Allow the mixture to cool slightly, around 5 minutes.

2. Take about 1/2 cup of the vegetable mixture and place it in the center of a warmed tortilla. Roll the tortilla over the filling and position the filled tortilla, seam-side down, in the prepared baking dish. Repeat this process with the remaining vegetable mixture and tortillas. Spread enchilada sauce over the tops of the enchiladas, then cover the baking dish with foil.

3. Bake until the sauce is bubbly, typically 15 to 20 minutes. Uncover and sprinkle with cheese; continue baking until the cheese is melted, approximately 5 minutes. If desired, garnish with cilantro before serving.

Tip: Store-bought enchilada sauce is a fast and easy way to add a ton of flavor to a dish, but it can be high in sodium, so look for one that has less than 300 milligrams sodium per serving.
Nutrition Information: Serving Size: 2 enchiladas
Calories 382, Fat 13g, Saturated Fat 5g, Cholesterol 19mg, Carbohydrates 52g, Total Sugars 6g, Added Sugars 0g, Protein 15g, Fiber 8g, Sodium 662mg, Potassium 498mg

Veggie Fajitas

Indulge in these veggie fajitas bursting with the sweetness of bell peppers and red onions. A delightful ensemble is achieved with creamy avocado and warm tortillas. The veggie mix itself is an excellent meal-prep option. Enjoy them over rice or heat them atop tortilla chips crowned with melted cheese. For that perfect char on your tortillas, place them over a medium gas flame until the spots darken, flipping once. Keep warm by covering them on a plate with a clean kitchen towel.

Active Time: 25 mins
Total Time: 25 mins
Servings: 6

Nutrition Notes:
Are Black Beans Healthy? Loaded with vitamins, minerals, antioxidants, and fiber, black beans enhance gut health, boost immunity, and reduce inflammation, reducing the risk of chronic diseases like heart disease and cancer. The fiber content may also help lower cholesterol and stabilize blood sugar.

Is Avocado Good for You? Avocados, rich in healthy fats, fiber, antioxidants, vitamins, and minerals, contribute to a healthful package associated with a lower rate of heart disease, improved brain function, and enhanced gut health. The monounsaturated fat in avocados, oleic acid, has been linked to decreased fat storage when consumed in adequate amounts.

What Vegetables Should I Use for Veggie Fajitas? Opt for multicolored bell peppers, red onions, and no-salt-added black beans. Feel free to introduce poblano peppers for a spicy kick and substitute no-salt-added pinto beans for black beans.

Can I Use Any Type of Tortillas for Veggie Fajitas? While corn tortillas are recommended for their robust flavor, you can use your preferred store-bought or homemade version. If you opt for flour tortillas, note that it will alter the recipe's nutritional profile.

Frequently Asked Questions:
What Can I Serve with Veggie Fajitas? Delight in veggie fajitas with warm corn tortillas or use the veggies for convenient meal prep. Serve them over Arroz Rojo Mexicano or Easy Cilantro-Lime Rice. Transform them into nachos by heating over tortilla chips with melted cheese. Pair veggie fajita nachos with Fresh Tomato Salsa, Copycat Chipotle Corn Salsa, or Roasted tomato salsa on the side.

Ingredients:
- 2 tablespoons extra-virgin olive oil
- 4 small multicolored bell peppers, thinly sliced
- 1 large red onion, thinly sliced
- 1 (15 ounce) can no-salt-added black beans, rinsed
- 2 tablespoons water
- 1 tablespoon ground cumin
- 1 tablespoon chili powder
- 2 teaspoons smoked paprika
- 1/2 teaspoon salt
- 1/2 teaspoon ground pepper
- 1/4 cup chopped fresh cilantro, plus cilantro leaves for garnish
- 1/4 cup lime juice
- 12 (6-inch) corn tortillas, warmed
- 1/3 cup crumbled cotija cheese
- 2 small avocados, thinly sliced

Instructions:
1. In a spacious nonstick skillet over medium-high heat, warm up the oil. Introduce bell peppers and onions, stirring occasionally, until they reach a delightful tenderness and a hint of char, typically around 12 minutes.

2. Next, incorporate black beans, water, cumin, chili powder, paprika, salt, and pepper. Keep stirring until the beans warm up and the spices generously coat the vegetables, roughly 4 minutes. Take it off the heat, then add cilantro and lime juice, giving it a final flavorful blend.

3. Now, portion out the mixture onto tortillas, generously topping them with cotija and avocado. For an extra touch, garnish with cilantro leaves if you fancy.

Nutrition Facts (per serving): 427 Calories / 23g Fat / 49g Carbs / 11g Protein

20-Minute Broccoli-Feta Soup

Crafted in just 20 minutes, this contemporary twist on classic cream of broccoli soup results in a velvety texture after a quick blender spin. Opt for pre-cut broccoli florets to expedite your prep, and pair this comforting soup with a delightful grilled cheese sandwich on the side for an indulgent dipping experience.

Active Time: 20 mins
Total Time: 20 mins
Servings: 4 servings

Ingredients:
- 2 tablespoons extra-virgin olive oil
- 1/2 cup thinly sliced scallions
- 3 cloves garlic, peeled and smashed
- 1 teaspoon dried basil
- 1/4 teaspoon crushed red pepper
- 4 cups reduced-sodium vegetable or chicken broth
- 1 pound broccoli crowns, stems and florets, cut into bite-size pieces (about 6 cups)
- 8 ounces Yukon Gold potatoes, scrubbed and cut into 1-inch pieces
- 1 tablespoon water
- 1/2 cup crumbled feta cheese, divided
- 1 teaspoon grated lemon zest, plus more for garnish
- 1/4 teaspoon salt

Instructions:
1. Begin by heating oil in a generously sized saucepan over medium-high heat. Introduce scallions, garlic, basil, and crushed red pepper; stir occasionally until the mixture turns bright green and emits a fragrant aroma, approximately 2 minutes. Pour in the broth and bring it to a boil over high heat. Add broccoli and continue stirring occasionally until it transforms into a vibrant green hue and becomes fork-tender, roughly 6 minutes.

2. Simultaneously, place potatoes and water in a medium microwave-safe bowl, covering it and microwaving on High until the potatoes achieve a very tender consistency, around 4 minutes.

3. Reserve 1 tablespoon of feta. Using a slotted spoon, transfer 1 cup of broccoli to a small bowl. Into the soup, stir the cooked potatoes, lemon zest, salt, and the remaining 7 tablespoons of feta. Transfer the entire concoction to a blender. Secure the blender lid and create a vent for steam by removing the center piece and covering the opening with a clean towel. Process until the mixture achieves a smooth consistency, taking approximately 1 minute. Exercise caution when blending hot liquids. Alternatively, you can use an immersion blender by removing the soup pot from heat and submerging the blender blades entirely under the liquid, pureeing until smooth for 3 to 5 minutes.

4. Distribute the soup evenly among 4 bowls. Spoon 1/4 cup of broccoli into each bowl and sprinkle with the reserved 1 tablespoon of feta and additional lemon zest for that finishing touch.

To make ahead: Refrigerate in an airtight container for up to 3 days.
Nutrition Information: Serving Size: 1 1/3 cups
Calories 200, Fat 10g, Saturated Fat 3g, Cholesterol 13mg, Carbohydrates 23g, Total Sugars 5g, Added Sugars 0g, Protein 8g, Fiber 5g, Sodium 470mg, Potassium 549mg

Heart-Healthy Recipes

One-Pot White Bean, Spinach & Sun-Dried Tomato Orzo with Lemon & Feta

Experience the lively and vibrant flavors of this one-pot pasta featuring white beans, spinach, and sun-dried tomatoes—a dish that not only delights your taste buds but also simplifies your cleanup. Elevating the orzo's taste with a quick toasting adds an extra layer of flavor to the mix. If you prefer, swap the spinach with another dark leafy green like chopped kale or Swiss chard, but keep in mind that sturdier greens may take a bit longer to wilt. If using a heartier green, add it to the pan during the last 5 minutes of cooking time.

Active Time: 25 mins
Total Time: 40 mins
Servings: 6 servings

Ingredients:
- 1 1/2 tablespoons extra-virgin olive oil
- 1 cup chopped red onion
- 6 cloves garlic, minced
- 1 cup whole-wheat orzo
- 1 cup chopped sun-dried tomatoes
- 2 3/4 cups vegetable broth
- 2 (15-ounce) cans no-salt-added cannellini beans, rinsed
- 1 teaspoon lemon zest
- 3 tablespoons lemon juice
- 3/4 teaspoon salt
- 1/2 teaspoon dried oregano
- 1 (5-ounce) package baby spinach
- 1/4 cup crumbled feta cheese
- 1/2 cup chopped fresh basil
- 1/4 cup toasted pine nuts

Instructions:
1. To begin, heat oil in a generously sized nonstick skillet over medium heat. Introduce the onion, stirring often until it becomes aromatic and translucent, typically around 8 minutes. Stir in the garlic, continuing to stir until it releases its aromatic essence, about 1 minute.

2. Now, incorporate the orzo and sun-dried tomatoes, ensuring to stir often until the orzo achieves a toasty perfection, roughly 1 minute. Add the broth, beans, lemon juice, salt, and oregano. Bring the mixture to a boil over medium-high heat. Once boiling, reduce the heat to medium-low, cover, and let it simmer until the orzo reaches an al dente consistency, approximately 15 minutes.

3. Stir in the spinach, and cook uncovered while stirring often until the spinach wilts, typically around 1 minute. Remove the skillet from heat and generously top the dish with feta, basil, pine nuts, and lemon zest for a delightful finish.

Nutrition Information: Serving Size: 1 cup
Calories 496, Fat 23g, Saturated Fat 1g, Cholesterol 4mg, Carbohydrates 60g, Total Sugars 14g, Added Sugars 0g, Protein 17g, Fiber 11g, Sodium 480mg, Potassium 895mg

Crispy Potato Latkes with Ikura

Honoring her Japanese roots, Maya Ono elevates these crispy latkes with a topping of ikura (salmon roe) and nori furikake, complemented by sour cream and scallions. However, feel free to customize the toppings to your liking. Opt for Russet potatoes as their starchiness aids in holding the latkes together.

Active Time: 1 hr 15 mins
Total Time: 1 hr 15 mins
Servings: 9 servings

Ingredients:
- 2 large russet potatoes, peeled
- 1/2 medium onion
- 1 1/2 tablespoons beaten egg (1/2 large) or liquid eggs
- 1 1/2 tablespoons all-purpose flour or matzo meal
- 1/2 teaspoon salt
- 1/4 teaspoon baking powder
- 1/2 cup grapeseed oil or other neutral oil or schmaltz (chicken or duck fat)
- 6 tablespoons sour cream or crème fraîche
- 3 tablespoons ikura (salmon roe)
- 6 tablespoons chopped scallions
- Nori furikake for garnish (optional)

Instructions:
1. Start by preheating the oven to 175°F (or the lowest oven temperature) and lining a baking sheet with paper towels.

2. On a cutting board, fold a large piece of cheesecloth in half. Grate the potatoes, one at a time, over the cheesecloth. After each potato, gather the cheesecloth to squeeze out the liquid and place the grated potato in a large bowl. Grate the onion onto the cheesecloth, squeeze out the liquid, and add the onion to the bowl with the potatoes.

3. To the potato mixture, add egg, flour (or matzo meal), salt, and baking powder. Mix until all the ingredients are well incorporated.

4. In a large skillet, preferably cast-iron, heat oil (or schmaltz) over medium-high heat. To check if the pan is ready, drop a small amount of batter; if it sizzles immediately, it's good to go. Spoon a heaping tablespoon of the potato mixture into the pan and flatten with a spatula, making 4 to 6 latkes for each batch. Cook the latkes, flipping once halfway, until deeply browned on both sides (approximately 3 to 5 minutes per side). Adjust the heat if needed to prevent burning. Transfer the latkes to the prepared baking sheet and keep them warm in the oven. Repeat the process with the remaining potato mixture.

5. Just before serving, top each latke with 1 teaspoon of sour cream and ½ teaspoon of ikura. Sprinkle with scallions and garnish with nori furikake if desired. Enjoy your personalized, delicious latkes!

Nutrition Information: Serving Size: 2 latkes
Calories 214, Fat 15g, Saturated Fat 2g, Cholesterol 23mg, Carbohydrates 18g, Total sugars 1g, Added sugars 0g, Protein 4g, Fiber 1g, Sodium 201mg, Potassium 380mg

Lemon-Garlic Salmon Bites

These marinated salmon bites are a speedy and delightful appetizer perfect for pleasing a crowd. While pink peppercorns add a touch of spice and a subtle floral note, freshly ground black peppercorns are a suitable alternative. Adjust the quantity accordingly, using just a quarter of black pepper due to its stronger flavor. Serve this appetizer with toothpicks alongside a light creamy dipping sauce, or transform it into a main dish on a bed of brown rice. Any leftovers can be repurposed to crown a green salad or tucked into pita bread with lettuce and tzatziki for an effortless sandwich.

Active Time: 15 mins
Total Time: 35 mins
Servings: 8 servings

Ingredients:
- 1 tablespoon grated lemon zest
- 3 tablespoons lemon juice
- 2 tablespoons extra-virgin olive oil
- 2 teaspoons grated garlic
- 1 teaspoon freshly ground pink peppercorns or 1/4 teaspoon ground black pepper, plus more for garnish
- 1 teaspoon salt, divided
- 1 pound center-cut salmon fillet, skinned and cut into 1-inch pieces
- 1 medium lemon, cut into 8 wedges (optional)
- 1 tablespoon chopped fresh flat-leaf parsley

Instructions:
1. In a medium nonreactive bowl, whisk together lemon zest, lemon juice, oil, garlic, ground pepper, and 3/4 teaspoon salt until emulsified, approximately 30 seconds. Add the salmon, tossing until evenly coated. Allow the salmon to marinate, uncovered, at room temperature for 15 minutes.

2. Preheat the broiler and position the oven rack 4 inches from the heat source. Line a broiler-safe baking sheet with foil. Arrange the marinated salmon pieces in a single layer on the prepared baking sheet, drizzling the remaining marinade over them. Sprinkle evenly with the remaining 1/4 teaspoon salt. If using, place lemon wedges on the baking sheet.

3. Broil until an instant-read thermometer inserted into the thickest portion registers 145°F, typically 5 to 7 minutes. Using tongs, transfer the salmon pieces to a serving platter. Squeeze the broiled lemon wedges over the salmon if desired. Sprinkle with parsley and garnish with additional ground pepper if you crave an extra kick. Enjoy the burst of flavors in this simple yet delectable dish!

Nutrition Facts (per serving): 152 Calories / 7g Fat / 12g Carbs / 13g Protein

High-Fiber Dragon Fruit & Pineapple Smoothie Bowl

This vibrant and high-fiber smoothie bowl is a feast for the eyes and the taste buds. Dragon fruit adds a burst of color without overpowering the other flavors, allowing them to shine. The combination of pineapple, pepitas, and bee pollen creates a visually stunning and delicious blend. The fizzy addition of kombucha lends a unique texture to this simple yet delightful smoothie bowl.

Active Time: 10 mins
Total Time: 25 mins

Servings: 1 serving

Ingredients:
- 1/3 cup unsweetened almond milk
- 2 tablespoons chia seeds
- 1 cup frozen pineapple chunks
- 3 ounces pink dragon fruit flesh (from about 1 pink-fleshed dragon fruit)
- 1/4 cup kombucha
- 1/4 cup sliced fresh pineapple
- 1 1/2 teaspoons unsalted raw pepitas
- 1 teaspoon bee pollen (optional)

Instructions:

1. In a serving bowl, whisk together almond milk and chia seeds. Allow it to chill until thickened, giving it a whisk after 7 minutes and letting it sit for a total of about 15 minutes.

2. In a blender, combine frozen pineapple, dragon fruit, and kombucha. Process on High until a smooth consistency is achieved, which typically takes about 1 minute.

3. Push the thickened chia mixture to one side of the bowl and pour the smoothie into the empty side. Top the bowl with sliced pineapple and pepitas. For an extra touch, sprinkle with bee pollen if desired. Enjoy this visually appealing and flavorful smoothie bowl!

Nutrition Facts (per serving): 314 Calories / 11g Fat / 52g Carbs / 8g Protein

Extra-Crispy Eggplant Parmesan

Indulge in this eggplant Parmesan featuring a creamy interior encased in a crispy panko crust. To ensure perfection, use the tip of a paring knife; it should effortlessly slide through the eggplant. If you encounter resistance, give it a few more minutes in the oven. Achieve even browning by rotating the baking sheet front to back.

Active Time: 30 mins
Total Time: 1 hr 15 mins
Servings: 4 serving

Ingredients:
- 1 medium eggplant, unpeeled
- 1 cup whole-wheat panko breadcrumbs
- 1/4 cup whole-wheat flour
- 1 large egg, lightly beaten
- 1 teaspoon salt-free Italian seasoning, such as Mrs. Dash
- 1/4 teaspoon garlic powder
- 1/4 teaspoon onion powder
- Cooking spray
- 1/4 teaspoon salt
- 1 cup lower-sodium marinara sauce
- 3/4 cup shredded low-moisture part-skim mozzarella cheese
- 1/4 cup grated Parmesan cheese

- 2 tablespoons extra-virgin olive oil
- Fresh basil leaves for garnish (optional)

Instructions:

1. Begin by preheating the oven to 425°F. Line a large-rimmed baking sheet with foil and set a wire rack on it. Cut the eggplant lengthwise into 4 slices, each ⅓-inch thick, while keeping the stem intact.

2. Prepare three wide, shallow bowls with panko, flour, and egg separately. Stir Italian seasoning, garlic powder, and onion powder into the panko.

3. Take one eggplant slice at a time, and dredge it in flour, shaking off excess. Dip it in egg, allowing excess to drip off. Coat it in the panko mixture, pressing to adhere, and place it on the prepared rack. Discard any leftover egg, flour, and panko.

4. Generously coat the tops of the eggplant slices with cooking spray. Bake until the panko becomes extra-crispy and browned, and the eggplant turns tender (approximately 40 minutes), remembering to flip and coat with cooking spray halfway through. Sprinkle with salt upon removal from the oven.

5. Boost the oven temperature to broil and preheat for 5 minutes. Top the eggplant slices with marinara, mozzarella, and Parmesan. Broil until the cheeses melt and acquire a golden brown hue in spots, lasting 2 to 3 minutes.

6. Distribute the eggplant slices among 4 plates, drizzling them with oil. If desired, garnish with basil. Savor the delightful combination of creamy insides and a crispy exterior in this delectable eggplant Parmesan!

Nutrition Facts (per serving): 307 Calories / 16g Fat / 30g Carbs / 12g Protein

Sweet Potato Home Fries with Cranberry-Hazelnut Crumble

Enjoy these sweet potato home fries, a fiber-rich and vitamin A-packed dish that supports a healthy immune system. For an extra touch of flavor, actor Anthony Anderson recommends adding a cranberry-hazelnut crumble.

Active Time: 25 mins
Total Time: 25 mins
Servings: 4 serving

Ingredients:
- 1 1/4 pounds sweet potatoes, cubed (1/2-inch)
- 1 teaspoon extra-virgin olive oil plus 1 tablespoon, divided
- 2 1/2 tablespoons chopped hazelnuts, toasted (see Tip)
- 2 tablespoons dried cranberries
- 1/8 teaspoon salt plus 1/4 teaspoon, divided
- 1/8 teaspoon ground pepper

Instructions:

1. Start by placing sweet potatoes in a large saucepan and covering them with water. Bring to a boil over high heat, then reduce to a simmer and cook until almost tender, approximately 6 to 8 minutes. Drain and pat dry with paper towels.

2. While the sweet potatoes are cooking, combine 1 teaspoon of oil, hazelnuts, cranberries, 1/8 teaspoon of salt, and pepper in a small bowl.

3. In a large cast-iron skillet, heat the remaining 1 tablespoon of oil over medium-high heat until it shimmers. Add the sweet potatoes and sprinkle with the remaining 1/4 teaspoon of salt. Allow them to cook for 3 minutes without stirring, then stir and continue cooking, stirring frequently, until crispy— about 5 minutes more. Transfer the home fries to a serving bowl and generously sprinkle them with the cranberry-hazelnut mixture. Delight in the upgraded and easy-to-make sweet potato home fries!

Tip: For the best flavor, toast nuts before using in a recipe. To toast chopped nuts, place in a small dry skillet and cook over medium-low heat, stirring constantly, until fragrant, 2 to 4 minutes.

Caramel Apple–Inspired Overnight Oats

Prepare this simple, meal-prep-friendly recipe that captures the essence of a caramel apple and transforms it into a delightful breakfast. The addition of applesauce ensures a creamy yet light texture, creating a perfect harmony with the sweet-tart flavor of the oats. If Granny Smith apples aren't available, feel free to use Fuji, Gala, or Honeycrisp apples as alternatives. Crushed honey-roasted peanuts mimic the coating of a caramel apple, though any salty-sweet nut will add deliciousness.

Active Time: 15 mins
Total Time: 8 hrs 15 mins
Servings: 4 serving
Ingredients:
- 2 cups old-fashioned rolled oats
- 2 cups unsweetened almond milk
- 2 cups chopped unpeeled Granny Smith apples, divided
- 1 cup unsweetened applesauce
- 2 tablespoons caramel sauce, divided
- 1 tablespoon plus 1 teaspoon chia seeds
- 2 teaspoons vanilla extract
- 2 teaspoons honey
- Chopped roasted peanuts, honey-roasted peanuts or glazed walnuts (optional)

Instructions:
1. In a medium bowl, combine oats, almond milk, 1 cup of apples, applesauce, 1 tablespoon of caramel sauce, chia seeds, vanilla, and honey. Stir until the mixture is evenly combined.

2. Spoon 1 cup of the mixture into each of the 4 (8-oz.) jars. Cover and refrigerate for at least 8 hours or up to 4 days.

3. When ready to serve, top each jar with 1/4 cup of apples and drizzle with 3/4 teaspoon of caramel sauce. Optionally, sprinkle with crushed nuts for an extra crunch. Enjoy this flavorful and convenient caramel apple-inspired breakfast!

To make ahead: Prepare through Step 2 and refrigerate for up to 4 days. Proceed with Step 3 when ready to serve.
Equipment: 4 (8-oz.) jars

Spicy Black-Eyed Pea & Collard Green Salad

This recipe for a black-eyed pea and collard green salad offers versatility, making it suitable for serving either warm or at room temperature. It works well as a side dish or serves as a satisfying vegetarian main course when paired with rice or crusty bread. Harissa and peri-peri sauce contribute a mild heat, while preserved lemon adds a briny tang.

Active Time: 45 mins
Total Time: 45 mins
Servings: 6 serving

Ingredients:
- 1 tablespoon neutral oil, such as grapeseed or canola
- 1 small shallot, chopped
- 1 clove garlic, thinly sliced
- ½ cup finely chopped yellow and/or red bell pepper
- 1 cup thinly sliced collard greens, coarsely chopped
- ½ teaspoon harissa paste (see Note)
- ¼ - ½ teaspoon peri-peri sauce (see Note)
- 2 cups cooked black-eyed peas or 1 15-ounce can no-salt-added black-eyed peas, rinsed
- ½ teaspoon turbinado sugar
- ¼ teaspoon sea salt
- ⅛ teaspoon ground pepper
- ¼ cup roughly chopped stemmed flat-leaf parsley
- 3 tablespoons extra-virgin olive oil
- 1 tablespoon lemon juice
- 1 tablespoon finely chopped preserved lemon
- 1 medium tomato, chopped

Instructions:
1. Begin by heating neutral oil in a medium skillet over medium heat. Add shallot and garlic, cooking and stirring until they become fragrant and slightly golden, typically 1 to 2 minutes. Introduce bell pepper, stirring occasionally until it begins to soften, about 1 to 3 minutes. Add collard greens, continuing to stir until they are slightly wilted, approximately 1 to 2 minutes. Incorporate harissa and peri-peri sauce, then mix in the black-eyed peas. Season with sugar, salt, and pepper. Reduce the heat to low and cook, stirring occasionally, for 3 to 5 minutes. Taste and adjust the seasoning if needed.

2. Transfer the mixture to a medium bowl. Add parsley, olive oil, lemon juice, and preserved lemon, ensuring a thorough mix. Fold in the tomato and adjust the seasoning if desired.

Notes: Harissa paste is a spicy North African condiment made with roasted chili peppers. Peri-peri (or piri-piri) sauce is a tangy hot sauce crafted from bird's eye chilies. Both can be found in well-stocked grocery stores or online. Note that heat levels vary among brands, so add a little at a time and taste as you go to achieve your preferred level of spiciness. If you choose to use only one, 3/4-1 tsp. of either harissa or peri-peri will suffice.

Healthy Low-Cholesterol Recipes

Roasted Honeynut Squash

Experience the delightful sweetness of honeynut squash, resembling mini butternut squash with its petite size and vibrant orange flesh. This straightforward roasting method, enriched with butter and spices, amplifies the natural flavors of the squash.

Prep Time: 10 mins
Additional Time: 30 mins
Total Time: 40 mins
Servings: 4
Yield: 4 servings

Nutrition Insights:
Is Honeynut Squash Nutrient-Rich?
Indeed, honeynut squash is a nutritional powerhouse akin to other winter squash varieties. Its deep orange hue indicates a high content of antioxidants, particularly beta-carotene, promoting eye health, immunity, and radiant skin. Packed with fiber, vitamin C, and potassium, honeynut squash also offers additional nutrition—protein, fiber, healthy fats, and more—by roasting the squash seeds.

Is This Recipe Suitable for Vegetarians?
Absolutely, as long as you include dairy, this recipe aligns with a vegetarian diet.

Test Kitchen Tips:
How to Best Cook Honeynut Squash?
Cooking honeynut squash mirrors the methods used for other winter squash varieties, but honeynut possesses unique advantages. Its modest size allows for easy halving, and its tender, edible skin eliminates the need for peeling. While you can steam, mash, or stuff honeynut squash, roasting it with minimal embellishments showcases its naturally sweet and nutty flavor.

Where Can I Find Honeynut Squash?
Discover honeynut squash in well-stocked grocery stores and farmers markets from September through December. Unlike some winter squash with longer shelf lives, honeynut squash is delicate and quickly loses its flavor, making it challenging to find out of season.

How to Prepare Honeynut Squash?
Each squash serves one to two people, offering a convenient size for quicker consumption. Here's a simple preparation guide:

Stabilize the squash on a cutting board and insert the tip of a large, heavy chef's knife into the center lengthwise. Use a folded kitchen towel for protection as you apply pressure to cut through one half, then rotate the squash 180 degrees and repeat.

Scoop out the seeds and the first shallow layer of flesh for a smoother surface. You can clean and roast the seeds, similar to pumpkin seeds, or discard them.

A preferred flavoring for honeynut squash involves a delightful combination of butter, cinnamon, salt, and pepper. Experiment with other flavor profiles if desired, but a general recommendation is around 1 teaspoon of butter or oil and a sprinkle of seasoning (approximately 1/4 teaspoon) per squash half.

Frequently Asked Questions:
What Is Honeynut Squash?
Honeynut squash, a newer hybrid of butternut squash, shares a similar shape but is much smaller,

approximately the size of a medium potato. Its vibrant orange skin mirrors the sweet and nutty flavor of its flesh.

In 2009, Chef Dan Barber challenged vegetable breeder Michael Mazourek to create a butternut squash with natural, delightful taste, reducing the need for added sugars like maple and honey. The result was the adorable honeynut squash, offering a sweeter butternut squash experience without additional sweeteners.

Ingredients:
- 2 medium honey nut squash, halved lengthwise and seeded
- 4 teaspoons butter
- ¼ teaspoon salt
- ¼ teaspoon ground pepper
- ¼ teaspoon ground cinnamon
- 4 teaspoons pure maple syrup (optional)

Instructions:
1. Preheat the oven to 425°F.

2. Next, lay the squash halves cut-side up on a spacious rimmed baking sheet. In each cavity, add 1 teaspoon of butter for a rich and indulgent touch. Sprinkle with a pinch of salt, a dash of pepper, and a hint of cinnamon to enhance the natural sweetness of the squash.

3. Roast the honeynut squash in the preheated oven until it becomes tender and irresistibly flavorful, typically taking 25 to 30 minutes.

4. For an extra layer of sweetness, drizzle each roasted squash half with maple syrup, if desired. This addition adds a delightful maple undertone that complements the innate sweetness of the honeynut squash, creating a harmonious and satisfying flavor profile.
5. Once the roasting is complete, your honeynut squash is ready to be enjoyed as a delectable side dish or a wholesome vegetarian main course. This simple yet flavorful recipe allows the natural characteristics of the honeynut squash to shine, offering a delightful culinary experience.

Nutrition Facts (per serving): 114 Calories / 4g Fat / 21g Carbs / 2g Protein

Maple-Roasted Sweet Potatoes

In this wholesome side dish, sweet potatoes undergo a delightful transformation as they are tossed with a mix of maple syrup, butter, and lemon juice, then roasted until achieving a tender, golden brown perfection. The resulting glaze elevates these maple-roasted sweet potatoes from a simple offering to a truly sublime culinary experience.

Prep Time: 10 mins
Additional Time: 1 hr
Total Time: 1 hr 10 mins
Servings: 12
Yield: 12 servings, about 1/2 cup each

Nutrition Insights:
Are Sweet Potatoes Beneficial to Your Health? Despite their name, sweet potatoes boast a low-glycemic

index and are brimming with essential vitamins, minerals, and fiber. Their combination of low-glycemic properties and fiber ensures they won't cause spikes in blood sugar levels. A medium-sized sweet potato delivers nearly 300% of your daily recommended intake of vitamin A, promoting healthy vision and supporting your immune system.

Is Maple Syrup a Healthy Choice? Pure maple syrup, extracted from the sap of the maple tree, can indeed be part of a healthy and diverse diet when consumed in moderation. It offers nutritional value, providing carbohydrates for energy and manganese, a mineral crucial for activating enzymes responsible for breaking down carbohydrates into usable fuel.

Test Kitchen Tips:
Should Sweet Potatoes be Peeled Before Roasting? While we peel the sweet potatoes in this recipe, you have the option to keep the skins on if you prefer a more textured experience. Sweet potato skins are edible, and leaving them on can also save you some prep time.

What Pan is Best for Roasting? Opt for a 9-by-13-inch baking dish to ensure the sweet potatoes roast evenly with ample depth for the delectable maple glaze. Cover the dish with foil during the initial 15 minutes of cooking to create a steaming effect, followed by uncovered roasting for an additional 45 to 50 minutes. Stir every 15 minutes to achieve the perfect balance of caramelization on the outside and tenderness on the inside.

Can Maple-Roasted Sweet Potatoes be Prepared in Advance? Certainly! After roasting, allow the sweet potatoes to cool completely, then store them in an airtight container in the refrigerator for up to three days. When ready to serve, reheat at 350°F until warmed through, approximately 15 to 20 minutes.

Frequently Asked Questions:
Which Sweet Potatoes are Suitable for this Recipe? Opt for an orange-flesh variety of sweet potatoes for this recipe, known for their denser and sweeter characteristics compared to the yellow-flesh variety. Common varieties include Beauregard, Jewel, and Garnet. Sweet potatoes are available year-round but are of the highest quality during the fall and early winter. Look for smooth-skinned sweet potatoes that are firm and free of soft spots, cracks, or bruises when selecting the best quality.

Ingredients:
- 2 ½ pounds sweet potatoes, peeled and cut into 1 1/2-inch pieces
- ⅓ cup pure maple syrup
- 2 tablespoons butter, melted
- 1 tablespoon lemon juice
- ½ teaspoon salt
- Freshly ground pepper, to taste

Instructions:
1. Preheat the oven to 400°F.

2. Now, arrange the sweet potatoes in a uniform layer within a 9-by-13-inch baking dish. In a small bowl, combine the maple syrup, butter, lemon juice, salt, and pepper to create a luscious glaze. Pour this delectable mixture over the sweet potatoes, ensuring each piece is thoroughly coated, and give them a gentle toss for an even distribution of flavors.

3. Cover the baking dish and let the sweet potatoes bake for the initial 15 minutes. Following this, uncover

the dish, stir the contents, and continue cooking, stirring every 15 minutes thereafter. This process ensures that the sweet potatoes become tender, develop a beautiful golden brown exterior, and absorb the irresistible flavors of the maple syrup, butter, and zesty lemon juice.

4. This roasting technique allows the sweet potatoes to reach the perfect balance of caramelization and tenderness. The result is a side dish that not only satisfies the taste buds but also showcases the natural sweetness and nutritional benefits of this vibrant root vegetable. Whether enjoyed as a comforting side or a nutritious main, these maple-roasted sweet potatoes are sure to become a beloved addition to your culinary repertoire.

Equipment: 9-by-13-inch baking dish
Nutrition Facts (per serving): 92 Calories / 2g Fat / 18g Carbs / 1g Protein

Black Bean Fajita Skillet

Streamline your dinner prep with the convenience of presliced fresh vegetables readily available in your grocer's produce section. Make the most of this time-saving option with a quick and easy Tex-Mex-inspired meal. In this recipe, pre-cut fajita vegetables are sautéed alongside canned black beans and Southwest seasoning, creating a flavorful and fuss-free dish. With just three main ingredients (excluding pantry staples like salt, pepper, and oil), you can have a delicious meal on the table in no time. Elevate your bowl by adding toppings such as cheese, sour cream, or other flavorful choices.

Active Time: 10 mins
Total Time: 15 mins
Servings: 2

Ingredients:
- 1 tablespoon olive oil
- 1 (12-ounce) package sliced fajita vegetables (bell peppers and onions)
- 1 (15-ounce) can no-salt-added black beans, rinsed
- ½ teaspoon salt-free Southwest-style seasoning blend
- ¼ teaspoon salt
- ¼ cup coarsely shredded Cheddar cheese (1 ounce; optional)

Instructions:
1. Begin by heating oil in a spacious skillet over medium heat. Sauté the presliced fajita vegetables until tender, a process that typically takes about 10 minutes.

2. Next, introduce the black beans, seasoning, and salt to the skillet. Cook and stir until the mixture is heated through, which typically takes around 1 minute.

3. Divide the vibrant and flavorful combination of vegetables and beans between two bowls. To enhance the experience, top each bowl with 2 tablespoons of cheese if desired.

4. This straightforward recipe allows you to enjoy a delicious and satisfying Tex-Mex-inspired meal with minimal effort. Feel free to customize your bowl with additional toppings of your choice, such as sour cream or other flavorful additions, for a personalized touch that suits your taste preferences.

Nutrition Facts (per serving): 310 Calories / 8g Fat / 47g Carbs / 14g Protein

Berry-Kefir Smoothie

Elevate your breakfast with a probiotic kick by incorporating kefir into your smoothie. This healthy and versatile smoothie recipe allows you to use any berries and nut butter you have available.

Prep Time: 5 mins
Total Time: 5 mins
Servings: 1
Yield: 1 serving

Ingredients:
- 1 ½ cups frozen mixed berries
- 1 cup plain kefir
- ½ medium banana
- 2 teaspoons almond butter
- ½ teaspoon vanilla extract

Instructions: In a blender, combine berries, kefir, banana, almond butter, and vanilla. Blend until the mixture reaches a smooth and creamy consistency. Enjoy a nourishing and flavorful start to your day!

Nutrition Facts (per serving): 304 Calories / 7g Fat / 53g Carbs / 15g Protein

Teriyaki Tofu Rice Bowls

In just 15 minutes, whip up a series of nutritious, high-fiber, and high-protein meals using convenient store-bought ingredients like pre-cooked rice packets and seasoned baked tofu.

Prep Time: 10 mins
Additional Time: 5 mins
Total Time: 15 mins
Servings: 4
Yield: 4 meal-prep containers
Ingredients:
- 2 (10 ounces) package cooked wild rice blend
- 1 tablespoon extra-virgin olive oil
- 1 (18-ounce) package of fresh Asian stir-fry vegetables
- 3 tablespoons teriyaki sauce
- 1 (7 ounces) package teriyaki-flavor baked tofu, cubed

Instructions:
1. Start by preparing the rice according to the package instructions. Transfer the cooked rice from the pouches to a shallow bowl, allowing it to cool.

2. In a medium nonstick skillet over medium heat, heat oil. Sauté the vegetables until they reach a crisp-tender texture, usually taking 4 to 5 minutes. Introduce teriyaki sauce to the mix, ensuring the vegetables are evenly coated. Remove from heat and set aside.

3. Divide the cooled rice among four single-serving containers. Layer each portion with a quarter of the sautéed vegetables, and distribute the tofu evenly among the containers. Seal the containers and refrigerate for up to 4 days. Before serving, vent the container and microwave until the contents are

steaming. Enjoy a quick, flavorful, and pre-prepared meal whenever you need it!

<u>To make ahead:</u> Refrigerate for up to 4 days.
<u>Nutrition Facts (per serving):</u> 360 Calories / 8g Fat / 59g Carbs / 15g Protein

Chopped Salad with Sriracha Tofu & Peanut Dressing

Prepare a week's worth of protein-packed vegan lunches effortlessly with just four simple ingredients from your local specialty grocery store. Begin with a robust veggie-heavy salad mix as your base, and if you can't find one, opt for broccoli slaw or shredded Brussels sprouts.

<u>Prep Time:</u> 10 mins
<u>Total Time:</u> 10 mins
<u>Servings:</u> 4
<u>Yield:</u> 4 servings

<u>Ingredients:</u>
- 1 (10 ounces) package of kale, Brussels sprout, broccoli, and cabbage salad mix
- 1 (12 ounces) package of frozen shelled edamame, thawed
- 2 (7 ounces) packages of Sriracha-flavored baked tofu, cubed
- 1/2 cup spicy peanut vinaigrette

<u>Instructions:</u>
1. Distribute the salad mix evenly among four single-serving containers with lids. On top of each, add 1/2 cup of edamame and a quarter of the tofu.

2. For added convenience, transfer 2 tablespoons of vinaigrette into each of four small lidded containers and refrigerate them for up to 4 days.

3. Seal the salad containers and store them in the refrigerator for a ready-to-go meal for up to 4 days. To enhance the flavors, dress the salad with vinaigrette up to 24 hours before serving. Enjoy a delicious and well-prepared vegan lunch with minimal effort.

<u>Tips:</u> To make ahead: Refrigerate for up to 4 days.
<u>Nutrition Facts (per serving):</u> 332 Calories / 15g Fat / 26g Carbs / 27g Protein

Seared Tuna with Bulgur & Chickpea Salad

Create a delightful and nutritious tuna dish by combining fresh fish, olive oil, lemon juice, herbs, and chickpeas. If you're cooking for two, repurpose the leftover tuna steaks by flaking them into the remaining bulgur salad. Serve this revitalizing salad over lettuce for a delightful lunch the next day.

<u>Prep Time:</u> 15 mins
<u>Additional Time:</u> 30 mins
<u>Total Time:</u> 45 mins
<u>Servings:</u> 4
<u>Yield:</u> 4 servings

<u>Ingredients:</u>
- ½ cup bulgur

- ¼ cup extra-virgin olive oil, divided
- 4 teaspoons grated lemon zest, divided
- ½ cup lemon juice, divided
- ½ teaspoon salt, divided
- ¼ teaspoon ground pepper
- 1 (15 ounces) can no-salt-added chickpeas
- ¼ cup chopped fresh Italian parsley
- ¼ cup chopped fresh mint
- 1 pound tuna, cut into 4 steaks (see Tip)
- 1 medium yellow onion, thinly sliced
- ¼ cup chopped fresh dill

Instructions:

1. Start by bringing a kettle of water to a boil. Place bulgur in a large heatproof bowl and add boiling water, ensuring it covers the bulgur by 2 inches. Let it stand for 30 minutes and then drain any excess water.

2. In a separate bowl, mix the soaked bulgur with 2 tablespoons of oil, 2 teaspoons of lemon zest, 1/4 cup of lemon juice, 1/4 teaspoon of salt, and pepper. Stir in chickpeas, parsley, and mint, ensuring an even combination. Set the bulgur salad aside.

3. In a large skillet over medium-high heat, heat the remaining 2 tablespoons of oil. Sear the tuna steaks until lightly browned on one side for 2 to 3 minutes, then flip and brown the other side. Transfer the tuna to a plate.

4. Reduce the heat to medium and add onions to the pan. Cook until translucent, approximately 5 minutes, stirring occasionally. Lower the heat to medium-low, return the tuna steaks to the pan, cover, and cook, flipping once, until the tuna flakes easily with a fork (slightly pink in the center), taking about 3 to 4 minutes per side.

5. While the tuna is cooking, combine dill with the remaining 1/4 cup of lemon juice and 1/4 teaspoon of salt in a small bowl.

6. Once the tuna is done, transfer it to a serving platter. Spoon the onions over the tuna and drizzle with the lemon juice-dill mixture. Sprinkle with the remaining 2 teaspoons of lemon zest and serve alongside the flavorful bulgur salad. Enjoy this healthy and delicious meal!

Tip: Ask at the seafood counter if your fishmonger can cut 1 lb. of tuna into four 4-oz. steaks.

To make ahead: Prepare bulgur (Step 1) and refrigerate for up to 2 days.

Nutrition Facts (per serving): 459 Calories / 16g Fat / 43g Carbs / 36g Protein

Chicken & Cucumber Lettuce Wraps with Peanut Sauce

Indulge in the delightful crunch of sliced cucumber and jicama in these delectable chicken lettuce wraps. Elevate the experience by serving them with a straightforward yet delicious peanut sauce, creating an impressive dinner recipe suitable for both kids and adults.

Prep Time: 40 mins
Total Time: 40 mins
Servings: 4
Yield: 8 lettuce wraps

Ingredients:
- ¼ cup creamy peanut butter
- 2 tablespoons low-sodium soy sauce
- 2 tablespoons honey
- 2 tablespoons water
- 2 teaspoons toasted sesame oil
- 2 teaspoons olive oil
- 3 scallions, sliced, white and green parts separated
- 1 serrano pepper, seeded and minced (2 tsp.)
- 1 tablespoon minced fresh ginger
- 2 teaspoons minced fresh garlic
- 1 pound ground chicken breast
- 1 cup diced jicama
- 16 Bibb lettuce leaves
- 1 cup cooked brown rice
- 1 cup halved and thinly sliced English cucumber
- ½ cup fresh cilantro leaves
- Lime wedges, for serving

Instructions:
1. In a small bowl, whisk together peanut butter, soy sauce, honey, water, and sesame oil.

2. Heat olive oil in a large nonstick skillet over medium heat. Add scallion whites, serrano, ginger, and garlic, cooking until they start to soften, approximately 2 minutes. Incorporate the chicken, breaking it up with a spoon or potato masher, and cook until fully cooked, which takes 3 to 4 minutes.

3. Introduce the peanut sauce to the chicken mixture, allowing it to thicken for about 3 minutes. Remove from heat and stir in jicama and scallion greens.

4. To serve, create 8 stacks of 2 lettuce leaves each. Fill the lettuce cups with rice, the chicken mixture, cucumber, and cilantro. Complete the experience by serving with lime wedges. Enjoy this easy and impressive meal!

Tips: Serves 4: 2 lettuce wraps each
Nutrition Facts (per serving): 521 Calories / 26g Fat / 44g Carbs / 34g Protein

Sweet Potato-Black Bean Burgers

Craft these delectable vegan sweet potato-black bean burgers infused with curry powder with ease. Achieve a soft, uniform texture by blending the mixture with your hands, while a crispy exterior is achieved through cooking in a cast-iron pan. For a gluten-free alternative, use gluten-free oats and opt for a lettuce wrap instead of a bun.

Prep Time: 15 mins
Additional Time: 30 mins
Total Time: 45 mins
Servings: 4
Yield: 4 burgers

Ingredients:
- 2 cups grated sweet potato
- ½ cup old-fashioned rolled oats
- 1 cup no-salt-added black beans, rinsed
- ½ cup chopped scallions
- ¼ cup vegan mayonnaise
- 1 tablespoon no-salt-added tomato paste
- 1 teaspoon curry powder
- ⅛ teaspoon salt
- 1/2 cup plain unsweetened almond milk yogurt
- 2 tablespoons chopped fresh dill
- 2 tablespoons lemon juice
- 2 tablespoons extra-virgin olive oil
- 4 whole-wheat hamburger buns, toasted
- 1 cup thinly sliced cucumber

Instructions:

1. Begin by squeezing grated sweet potato with paper towels to eliminate excess moisture, then place it in a large bowl. In a food processor, pulse oats until finely ground and add them to the bowl with the sweet potatoes. Introduce beans, scallions, mayonnaise, tomato paste, curry powder, and salt to the bowl; use your hands to mash the mixture together. Shape it into four 1/2-inch-thick patties and refrigerate on a plate for 30 minutes.

2. Prepare a yogurt sauce by stirring together yogurt, dill, and lemon juice in a small bowl; set it aside.

3. Heat oil in a large cast-iron skillet over medium-high heat. Cook the patties until golden brown, approximately 3 minutes per side.

4. For assembly, evenly distribute the yogurt sauce on the top and bottom halves of the bun. Place a burger and cucumber slices on each bottom bun half and replace the top bun halves. Relish in these flavorful burgers, embracing the delightful combination of sweet potato and black beans.

Tips: To make ahead: Prepare patties (Step 1); wrap and refrigerate for up to 2 days.
Nutrition Facts (per serving): 454 Calories / 22g Fat / 54g Carbs / 12g Protein

Bone-Health Recipes

Spinach & Mushroom Quiche

Discover the simplicity of this healthy vegetarian quiche, where the fuss of a traditional crust is left behind. Brimming with the sweetness of wild mushrooms and the savory richness of Gruyère cheese, this dish is a delightful choice for breakfast, brunch, or a light lunch when accompanied by a fresh salad.

Active Time: 25 mins
Total Time: 1 hr 5 mins
Servings: 6
Yield: 1 quiche

Nutrition Insights:
Once a point of contention due to cholesterol concerns, eggs are now embraced by health experts, with

the American Heart Association approving an egg a day as part of a balanced diet. Loaded with protein, eggs, especially the yolk, offer essential nutrients like iron, vitamin B12, and choline. Furthermore, nearly half of your daily vitamin D needs can be met with just two large eggs.

Mushrooms, with their earthy goodness, provide niacin, a B vitamin crucial for energy metabolism. These fungi also offer a dose of plant-based protein and boast compounds that support the gut, bolster the immune system, and potentially reduce cancer risk. Recent research even suggests that exposing mushrooms to ultraviolet light can enhance their vitamin D content, addressing a common deficiency.

Gluten-Free and Vegetarian Delight: This recipe caters to gluten-free and vegetarian preferences, making it an inclusive and satisfying option for various dietary needs.

Insights from the Test Kitchen:
For those without sweet onions, a white or yellow onion can be a suitable substitute. While sweet onions are preferred for their milder flavor, the alternative onions provide a mild taste when cooked.

Frozen spinach can seamlessly replace fresh spinach, provided it is thawed and well-drained. To prevent a watery quiche, ensure that any fresh or frozen veggies are adequately squeezed dry or pre-cooked before incorporating them into the custard.

In the absence of half-and-half, whole milk can step in as a viable alternative. While this may result in a slightly less creamy texture, the overall flavor remains intact.

Cheese Swaps: Gruyère cheese, originating from Switzerland, adds a mild, nutty flavor and creamy texture that complements the quiche beautifully. However, if you prefer variety, feel free to substitute it with Swiss, Gouda, or Cheddar for an alternative twist.

Prepare in Advance: This quiche is versatile enough to be made ahead of time, offering the convenience of refrigerating it for up to 5 days. When ready to enjoy, either reheat the entire quiche at 350°F for 30 to 45 minutes or opt for a slice-by-slice reheating in the microwave.

Ingredients:
- 2 tablespoons extra-virgin olive oil
- 8 ounces sliced fresh mixed wild mushrooms such as cremini, shiitake, button and/or oyster mushrooms
- 1 ½ cups thinly sliced sweet onion
- 1 tablespoon thinly sliced garlic
- 5 ounces fresh baby spinach (about 8 cups), coarsely chopped
- 6 large eggs
- ¼ cup whole milk
- ¼ cup half-and-half
- 1 tablespoon Dijon mustard
- 1 tablespoon fresh thyme leaves, plus more for garnish
- ¼ teaspoon salt
- ¼ teaspoon ground pepper
- 1 ½ cups shredded Gruyère cheese

Instructions:
1. Begin by preheating the oven to 375°F and coating a 9-inch pie pan with cooking spray.

2. In a large nonstick skillet set over medium-high heat, heat oil and sauté mushrooms until browned and tender, approximately 8 minutes. Add onions and garlic, continuing to cook until softened and tender (about 5 minutes). Introduce spinach and toss continuously until wilted (1 to 2 minutes). Remove the mixture from heat.

3. In a medium bowl, whisk together eggs, milk, half-and-half, mustard, thyme, salt, and pepper. Gently fold in the mushroom mixture and cheese. Spoon the mixture into the prepared pie pan.

4. Bake until the quiche is set and golden brown, typically around 30 minutes. Allow it to stand for 10 minutes before slicing. Garnish with additional thyme and serve this delectable Spinach & Mushroom Quiche.

Equipment: 9-inch pie pan, large nonstick skillet.
Nutrition Facts (per serving): 277 Calories / 20g Fat / 7g Carbs / 17g Protein

Air-Fryer Salmon Cakes

Reminiscent of classic salmon croquettes, these air-fried salmon patties offer a delightful combination of a crispy exterior and a tender, pillowy interior. Look for canned or jarred salmon with less than 50 milligrams of sodium per serving, and don't shy away from varieties containing bones—they're easy to remove.

Active Time: 10 mins
Additional Time: 15 mins
Total Time: 25 mins
Servings: 2
Yield: 4 cakes

Air-Fryer Salmon Cake Preparation: Harnessing the convenience of canned salmon, these air-fryer salmon cakes are a quick and easy pantry staple creation. The air fryer imparts a satisfying crispiness to the outer layer, using significantly less oil than stovetop alternatives. Here's a step-by-step guide:

Prep with Cooking Spray: Utilize cooking spray to coat the air fryer basket, preventing the salmon cakes from sticking. Give your salmon cakes another light spray once they're in the basket.

Mixing the Ingredients: This uncomplicated recipe combines canned salmon with egg, panko breadcrumbs, fresh dill, mayonnaise, Dijon mustard, and pepper. Before blending, sift through the canned salmon, discarding any large bones. Smaller bones and skin are edible and provide additional calcium. Mix the ingredients gently, shaping the mixture into four 3-inch patties.

Air-Frying the Salmon Cakes: Once the patties are formed, they're ready for the air fryer. Depending on your air fryer's size, you might need to cook them in batches. Overcrowding the basket hinders airflow, resulting in less crispiness. For batch cooking, transfer the first batch to a baking sheet, keeping them warm in a 200°F oven while the second batch cooks. Cook the patties in a 400°F air fryer until browned, and an instant-read thermometer reads 160°F in the thickest portion, approximately 12 minutes.

Serving Suggestions for Air Fryer Salmon Cakes: These salmon patties shine on their own, adorned with a squeeze of lemon juice. Alternatively, elevate them by incorporating them into a salad, pita bread, or on a hamburger bun. Consider enhancing the experience with a creamy spread featuring capers, dill, parsley, or cucumber.

Ingredients:
- Cooking spray
- 2 7.5-ounce cans of unsalted pink salmon (with skin and bones)
- 1 large egg
- ½ cup whole-wheat panko breadcrumbs
- 2 tablespoons chopped fresh dill
- 2 tablespoons canola mayonnaise
- 2 teaspoons Dijon mustard
- ¼ teaspoon ground pepper
- 2 lemon wedges

Instructions:
1. Prepare the Air Fryer: Coat the air fryer basket with cooking spray.

2. Prep the Salmon: Drain the salmon and discard any large bones and skin. Place the salmon in a medium bowl. Add egg, panko, dill, mayonnaise, mustard, and pepper. Gently stir until well combined. Shape the mixture into four 3-inch-diameter cakes.

3. Air-Fry the Salmon Cakes: Coat the cakes with cooking spray and place them in the prepared basket. Air fry at 400°F until browned, and an instant-read thermometer inserted into the thickest portion registers 160°F, approximately 12 minutes.

4. Serve with Lemon Wedges: Present the air-fried salmon cakes with lemon wedges for a delightful finishing touch.

Nutrition Facts (per serving): 517 Calories / 27g Fat / 15g Carbs / 52g Protein

Eggplant Parmesan

Revitalize your Eggplant Parmesan with this healthier, baked version that retains the crispy appeal while cutting down on calories.

Cook Time: 20 mins
Active Time: 25 mins
Total Time: 45 mins
Servings: 6
Yield: 6 servings

Ingredients:
- Canola or olive oil cooking spray
- 2 large eggs
- 2 tablespoons water
- 1 cup panko breadcrumbs
- ⅓ cup grated Parmesan cheese, divided
- 1 teaspoon Italian seasoning
- 2 medium eggplants (about 2 pounds total), cut crosswise into ¼-inch-thick slices
- ½ teaspoon salt
- ½ teaspoon ground pepper
- 1 (24 ounces) jar of no-salt-added tomato sauce

- ¼ cup fresh basil leaves, torn, plus more for serving
- 2 cloves garlic, grated
- ½ teaspoon crushed red pepper
- 1 cup shredded part-skim mozzarella cheese, divided

Creating a Healthier Eggplant Parmesan:
Eggplant Parmesan, a timeless comfort dish, becomes a wholesome delight with a few adjustments. Our rendition features tender eggplant, a crunchy crust, flavorful tomato sauce, and a generous layer of cheese—all reminiscent of the classic version but with reduced calories, less fat, and lower sodium content. Here's the breakdown:

Ditch the Frying: The typical crispy crust on eggplant Parmesan often involves breading and frying slices in oil. While we cherish that crispy texture, our approach achieves the same results with a healthier twist. After breading the eggplant slices, we opt for a baking method—spraying them with cooking spray and baking in the oven. This technique ensures a light, even coating of oil, preserving the crispy breading while significantly cutting down on fat and calories.

Elevate the Tomato Sauce: An excellent Eggplant Parmesan hinges on a rich tomato sauce, crucial for keeping the eggplant moist during baking. Traditional tomato sauces can be high in sodium, potentially impacting blood pressure. To mitigate this, our recipe embraces no-salt-added tomato sauce. To enhance flavor without relying on salt, we introduce fresh basil, garlic, and crushed red pepper into the sauce, ensuring a robust taste that compensates for the reduced sodium.

Opt for Flavorful Cheese Pairing: Achieving the sought-after ooey-gooey cheese factor in Eggplant Parmesan is key, and we do this smartly. Choosing part-skim mozzarella over whole-milk mozzarella maintains a silky texture while minimizing saturated fat. With sodium savings from the no-salt-added tomato sauce, we enrich the cheese layer by incorporating Parmesan. This addition strategically brings savory depth without compromising on flavor.

Indulge in the revamped goodness of this healthier Eggplant Parmesan, where every bite is a fusion of crispy satisfaction and mindful nutrition.

Instructions:
1. Prepare for Baking: Position racks in the middle and lower thirds of the oven, preheating to 400°F. Coat two baking sheets and a 9-by-13-inch baking dish generously with cooking spray, ensuring a non-stick surface for your delicious Eggplant Parmesan.

2. Breading and Baking the Eggplant: In a shallow bowl, whisk together eggs and water. In another shallow dish, combine breadcrumbs, 1/4 cup Parmesan, and Italian seasoning. Dip each eggplant slice in the egg mixture, then coat it with the breadcrumb mixture, gently pressing to ensure adhesion. Arrange the breaded eggplant in a single layer on the prepared baking sheets. Generously spray both sides with cooking spray. Bake for approximately 30 minutes, flipping the eggplant and switching the pans between racks halfway through. The result: tender, lightly browned eggplant slices. Season with salt and pepper for the perfect finish.

3. Prepare the Tomato Sauce: While the eggplant is baking, mix together tomato sauce, basil, garlic, and crushed red pepper in a medium bowl. This flavorful sauce will complement the crispy eggplant beautifully.

4. Assemble the Layers: Begin assembling your Eggplant Parmesan layers. Spread about 1/2 cup of the prepared sauce in the baking dish. Arrange half of the baked eggplant slices over the sauce, followed by another cup of sauce. Sprinkle 1/4 cup Parmesan and 1/2 cup mozzarella over the sauce. Repeat the layering process with the remaining eggplant, sauce, and cheese.

5. Final Baking: Bake the assembled dish until the sauce is bubbling and the top achieves a golden hue, usually taking 20 to 30 minutes. Once done, allow it to cool for 5 minutes, allowing the flavors to meld and the layers to set.

6. Finishing Touch: Before serving, sprinkle additional basil over the top for a fresh and aromatic garnish. This step adds a burst of color and a final layer of herbaceous flavor to your wonderfully revamped, healthier Eggplant Parmesan.

Nutrition Facts (per serving): 241 Calories / 9g Fat / 28g Carbs / 14g Protein

Cucumber-Yogurt Salad

A delightful companion to meat or fish dishes, this cucumber-yogurt salad also transforms into a flavorful filling for pita bread. Grate the cucumbers for a unique dip variation.

Active Time: 20 mins
Total Time: 20 mins
Servings: 4
Yield: 4 servings

Nutrition Insights:
Cucumbers: Containing about 95% water, cucumbers are a hydrating vegetable with antioxidants that may aid in preventing the multiplication of cancer cells. The presence of minerals, particularly silica, contributes to skin nourishment, promoting smoothness and firmness. Additionally, cucumbers are known to potentially assist in preventing diabetes.

Yogurt: A nutritional powerhouse, yogurt serves as an excellent protein source loaded with calcium, phosphorous, and vitamin B12. Rich in potassium, zinc, and vitamin D, yogurt supports bone and muscle growth, a robust nervous and immune system, cell growth and development, and healthy blood pressure. The probiotics in yogurt enhance digestion by introducing beneficial bacteria to the gut's microbiome.

Test Kitchen Tips:
Choosing Cucumbers: Opt for American cucumbers, labeled simply as "cucumber" in grocery stores, with thicker skin. These cucumbers, specifically Americana Slicing Hybrid, have larger seeds, typically scooped out to eliminate excess moisture in various dishes.

Fresh Herb Options: Feel free to personalize your salad with a variety of fresh herbs. In addition to parsley and mint, consider incorporating dill or chives for an extra burst of flavor.

Making Ahead: While you can prepare the yogurt mixture in advance and refrigerate it for up to one day in an airtight container, we recommend assembling the cucumber yogurt salad on the day of serving. Cucumbers release moisture over time, and making it ahead may result in an overly watery consistency.

FAQs:
Peeling Cucumbers: For American cucumbers, it's advisable to peel their tougher skin, often coated in

wax. Thin-skinned varieties like English or Persian cucumbers do not require peeling.

Preventing Sogginess: To maintain cucumber crispness, lightly salt the slices for at least 20 minutes, drawing out excess moisture. Removing seeds and pulp further prevents sogginess in salads, ensuring a crisp texture. The salt not only aids in moisture removal but also lightly seasons the cucumbers before adding the yogurt mixture.

Ingredients:
- 4 large cucumbers, peeled
- ½ teaspoon salt
- 2 cups low-fat plain yogurt
- 2 teaspoons lemon juice
- 2-4 cloves garlic, minced
- Freshly ground pepper, to taste
- 2 tablespoons chopped fresh parsley, or 2 tablespoons chopped fresh mint
- 1 tablespoon extra-virgin olive oil

Instructions:
1. Prepare Cucumbers: Begin by cutting the cucumbers in half and removing the seeds. Cut each cucumber boat in half lengthwise, then halve each quarter, creating bite-sized pieces. Crosswise, slice the cucumber into 1/4-inch pieces. Place the cucumber slices in a bowl, sprinkle salt on top, toss them gently, and set aside for at least 20 minutes. This step draws out excess moisture, ensuring the cucumbers maintain a delightful crispness.

2. Create the Yogurt Mixture: In a separate medium bowl, combine yogurt, lemon juice, garlic, pepper, and either parsley or mint, depending on your preference. Stir in the oil briskly to achieve a well-blended, flavorful yogurt mixture. This combination of ingredients adds a zesty and aromatic touch to complement the coolness of the cucumbers.

3. Drain and Assemble: After the 20-minute resting period, drain the cucumbers to eliminate the excess liquid. Return the drained cucumbers to the bowl and pour the prepared yogurt mixture over them. Toss the ingredients well to ensure every cucumber piece is coated with the refreshing yogurt blend. This vibrant mixture combines the hydrating qualities of cucumbers with the creamy texture of yogurt, creating a harmonious balance of flavors and textures.

4. Serve and Enjoy: Your cucumber-yogurt salad is now ready to be served alongside your favorite main course or as a delightful pita bread filling. The combination of crisp cucumbers and the tangy yogurt mixture offers a refreshing and health-conscious addition to your meal. Garnish with additional fresh herbs or a sprinkle of black pepper for an extra burst of flavor, if desired.

Nutrition Facts (per serving): 146 Calories / 6g Fat / 16g Carbs / 8g Protein

Pesto Ravioli with Spinach & Tomatoes

Savor the simplicity of this swift ravioli recipe featuring just five ingredients yet bursting with vibrant flavors. With the convenience of grape tomatoes, prewashed spinach, and ready-made pesto, this Caprese-inspired dish is the ultimate weeknight meal, taking only 15 minutes from start to finish.

Prep Time: 15 mins

Total Time: 15 mins
Servings: 4
Yield: 5 cups

Choosing Your Ingredients: For this fuss-free weeknight delight, all you need are five readily available ingredients. Here are some guidelines for a seamless shopping experience:

Selecting the Ravioli: Opt for frozen or refrigerated cheese ravioli, typically filled with a delightful blend of ricotta, mozzarella, and Parmesan cheese. Some variations may even feature a combination of four or five cheeses. Choose your preferred brand, keeping an eye on sodium levels. Aim for entrees with 480 milligrams or less of sodium for a heart-conscious choice.

Choosing the Pesto: Whether homemade or store-bought, the pesto choice is yours. For store-bought pesto that mirrors a homemade taste, explore options in the refrigerated section. If opting for shelf-stable jarred pesto, seek out a brand with a vibrant green hue and minimal oil content.

Ingredients:
- 2 8-ounce packages frozen or refrigerated cheese ravioli
- 1 tablespoon olive oil
- 1 pint grape tomatoes
- 1 5-ounce package baby spinach
- ⅓ cup pesto

Instructions:
1. Boil the Ravioli: Bring a large pot of water to a boil. Cook the ravioli according to package instructions, drain, and set aside.

2. Sauté the Tomatoes: In a spacious nonstick skillet over medium heat, heat oil. Add grape tomatoes and sauté until they begin to burst, a delightful process taking around 3 to 4 minutes.

3. Add Spinach: Introduce prewashed spinach to the skillet, stirring frequently until it gently wilts, usually 1 to 2 minutes.

4. Combine with Ravioli and Pesto: Incorporate the cooked ravioli into the skillet, along with the pesto. Gently stir to combine all the elements, ensuring the flavors meld seamlessly.

Equipment: Large nonstick skillet
Nutrition Facts (per serving): 361 Calories / 19g Fat / 35g Carbs / 14g Protein

Turkey Burgers with Spinach, Feta & Tzatziki

Elevate your burger experience with the refreshing flavors of creamy tzatziki and crisp cucumber, complementing a delightful combination of feta and spinach in this effortless recipe. Don't have tzatziki? Not an issue! Create your own at home by blending plain strained yogurt with a dash of lemon, dill, and finely chopped cucumber.

Prep Time: 30 mins
Total Time: 30 mins
Servings: 4
Yield: 4 burgers

Ingredients:
- 1 cup frozen chopped spinach, thawed
- 1 pound 93% lean ground turkey
- ½ cup crumbled feta cheese
- ½ teaspoon garlic powder
- ½ teaspoon dried oregano
- ¼ teaspoon salt
- ¼ teaspoon ground pepper
- 4 small hamburger buns, preferably whole-wheat, split
- 4 tablespoons tzatziki
- 12 slices cucumber
- 8 thick rings of red onion (about 1/4 inch)

Instructions:
1. Preheat the Grill: Start by preheating the grill to medium-high heat, ensuring it's ready for the grilling action.

2. Prepare the Spinach Turkey Blend: Remove excess moisture from the spinach, then combine it with ground turkey, feta, garlic powder, oregano, salt, and pepper in a medium bowl. Ensure a thorough mix to distribute the flavors evenly. Shape the mixture into four 4-inch patties.

3. Grill the Patties: Prevent sticking by oiling the grill rack. Grill the patties until they are fully cooked, achieving a lovely golden exterior. This generally takes about 4 to 6 minutes per side. Confirm their readiness by using an instant-read thermometer, ensuring the center registers 165°F.

4. Burger Assembly: Assemble the burgers by placing the cooked patties on your preferred buns. Enhance each burger by topping it with a generous tablespoon of tzatziki, three cucumber slices, and two rings of onion. This final touch adds a burst of freshness and texture.

To make ahead: Prepare patties, wrap individually and refrigerate for up to 8 hours.
Tip: To oil a grill rack, oil a folded paper towel, hold it with tongs and rub it over the rack. (Do not use cooking spray on a hot grill.)

Nutrition Facts (per serving): 376 Calories / 17g Fat / 29g Carbs / 30g Protein

Mozzarella, Basil & Zucchini Frittata

This frittata recipe, brimming with colorful vegetables, is a speedy and versatile meal that can grace your breakfast table or elevate lunch and dinner when paired with a crisp salad and a slice of crusty baguette drizzled with olive oil.

Cook Time: 20 mins
Total Time: 20 mins
Servings: 4
Yield: 4 servings

Ingredients:
- 2 tablespoons extra-virgin olive oil
- 1 ½ cups thinly sliced red onion
- 1 ½ cups chopped zucchini

- 7 large eggs, beaten
- ½ teaspoon salt
- ¼ teaspoon freshly ground pepper
- ⅔ cup pearl-size or baby fresh mozzarella balls (about 4 ounces)
- 3 tablespoons chopped soft sun-dried tomatoes
- ¼ cup thinly sliced fresh basil

Instructions:

1. Preheat the Broiler: Set the oven rack in the upper third position and preheat the broiler for optimal results.

2. Sauté Vegetables: Heat oil in a large broiler-safe nonstick or cast-iron skillet over medium-high heat. Add diced onion and zucchini, stirring frequently until they become tender, a process taking around 3 to 5 minutes.

3. Prepare the Eggs: While the vegetables cook, whisk together eggs, salt, and pepper in a bowl. Once the vegetables are soft, pour the whisked eggs over them in the skillet. Cook, gently lifting the edges to let the uncooked egg flow underneath, until the frittata is nearly set—this typically takes about 2 minutes.

4. Add Toppings and Broil: Sprinkle mozzarella and sun-dried tomatoes on top of the partially set eggs. Place the skillet under the broiler until the eggs achieve a delightful slight browning, usually 1 1/2 to 2 minutes.

5. Let It Rest: Allow the frittata to stand for 3 minutes, allowing the flavors to meld. Top it off with fresh basil for an extra burst of freshness.

6. Serve with Ease: To release the frittata from the pan, gently run a spatula around the edges and underneath. Once loosened, slide or lift it onto a cutting board or serving plate. Slice it into 4 equal portions and serve promptly.

Nutrition Facts (per serving): 292 Calories / 21g Fat / 8g Carbs / 18g Protein

Creamy Radish Soup

Delight in the creamy goodness of this radish soup, where sautéed radishes join forces with potatoes to create a velvety and nourishing delight. The cooking process mellows the radishes' bitterness, leaving behind a blend of sweet and earthy flavors. Opt for smaller radishes for a charming pink hue, while larger ones yield an almost white soup.

Cook Time: 30 mins
Total Time: 30 mins
Servings: 4
Yield: 4 servings

Ingredients:
- 2 tablespoons extra-virgin olive oil
- 2 cups sliced radishes (from 2 bunches), divided
- ½ cup chopped onion
- 1 medium Yukon Gold potato (about 8 ounces), peeled and cut into 1-inch cubes
- 2 cups low-fat milk

- ½ teaspoon salt
- 1/4-1/2 teaspoon white or black pepper
- ¼ cup reduced-fat sour cream
- 1 tablespoon chopped fresh radish greens or parsley

Instructions:
1. Sauté Radishes and Onions: Heat oil in a sizable saucepan over medium-high heat. Add 1 3/4 cups of radishes and onions, stirring frequently until the onions begin to brown and the radishes turn translucent, typically around 5 minutes.

2. Add Potato and Milk: Introduce potato, milk, salt, and pepper to the saucepan, stirring occasionally. Bring the mixture to a gentle boil. Once boiling, reduce the heat to a simmer, cover, and cook, stirring occasionally, until the potato achieves tenderness—approximately 5 minutes more.

3. Puree the Mixture: With caution due to the hot liquid, puree the mixture in batches using a blender or use an immersion blender directly in the pan until the consistency is smooth.

4. Garnish and Serve: Slice the remaining 1/4 cup of radishes into matchsticks. Serve each portion of the soup topped with 1 tablespoon of sour cream, a generous sprinkle of radish matchsticks, and a touch of radish greens or parsley for a finishing touch.

Tips: Make Ahead Tip: Cover and refrigerate for up to 3 days.
Nutrition Facts (per serving): 203 Calories / 10g Fat / 22g Carbs / 6g Protein

Vegetarian Spaghetti Squash Lasagna

Experience a low-carb twist on traditional lasagna with these delightful spaghetti squash lasagna boats. Layers of savory mushrooms, tomato sauce, and spaghetti squash noodles create a satisfying dish. Crafted right within the spaghetti squash shells, topped with melted mozzarella for a gooey finish, these boats promise both a visually appealing presentation and a healthy dinner option. Complete the meal with a crisp green salad and a glass of Chianti.

Prep Time: 50 mins
Additional Time: 20 mins
Total Time: 1 hr 10 mins
Servings: 4
Yield: 4 servings

Ingredients:
- 1 2 1/2- to 3-pound spaghetti squash, halved lengthwise and seeded
- ¼ cup water
- 2 tablespoons extra-virgin olive oil
- 1 medium onion, chopped
- 4 cloves garlic, minced
- 10 ounces mushrooms, sliced
- 2 cups crushed tomatoes
- 1 teaspoon Italian seasoning
- ½ teaspoon ground pepper, divided
- ¼ teaspoon crushed red pepper
- ¼ teaspoon salt, divided

- ¼ cup grated Parmesan cheese
- 1 cup shredded part-skim mozzarella cheese, divided
- ½ cup part-skim ricotta cheese

Instructions:

1. Preheat the Oven: Position the oven rack in the upper third and preheat to 450 degrees F.

2. Prepare the Spaghetti Squash: Place the spaghetti squash cut-side down in a microwave-safe dish with water. Microwave on High until the flesh is tender, approximately 10 to 12 minutes. Alternatively, bake the squash cut-side down on a large rimmed baking sheet at 400 degrees F until tender, about 40 to 50 minutes.

3. Sauté Vegetables: In a large skillet over medium heat, heat oil and sauté onions and garlic until soft, around 3 to 4 minutes. Add mushrooms and continue cooking until the vegetables are tender and lightly browned about 5 minutes. Stir in tomatoes, Italian seasoning, 1/4 teaspoon pepper, crushed red pepper, and 1/8 teaspoon salt. Cook until heated through and flavors meld, about 1 to 2 minutes. Remove from heat and cover.

4. Prepare Squash Mixture: Use a fork to scrape the spaghetti squash from the shells into a large bowl. Stir in Parmesan, remaining 1/4 teaspoon pepper, and remaining 1/8 teaspoon salt.

5. Assemble the Lasagna Boats: Place the squash shells cut-side up on a large rimmed baking sheet. Spoon one-fourth of the squash-Parmesan mixture into each shell. Layer one-fourth of the tomato mixture on top, then sprinkle 1/4 cup mozzarella into each shell. Dollop 1/4 cup ricotta over the mozzarella. Repeat the layering with the remaining squash mixture, tomato sauce, and mozzarella.

6. Bake and Broil: Bake the squash lasagna boats for 15 minutes. Turn the broiler to high and broil, keeping a close eye, until the cheese starts to brown, approximately 1 to 2 minutes.

Nutrition Facts (per serving): 350 Calories / 18g Fat / 34g Carbs / 18g Protein

Healthy Pregnancy Recipes

4-Ingredient Adas bis-Silq (Lentil & Chard Soup)

Even with just a handful of ingredients, this lentil soup packs a punch of flavor. A drizzle of special olive oil and the option to substitute chard with kale or collards make it a versatile delight. The following is an excerpt from "Lebanese Cuisine" by Madelain Farah and Leila Habib-Kirske, published by Hatherleigh Press.

Active Time: 25 mins
Total Time: 45 mins
Servings: 6

Ingredients:
- 6 cups water
- 1 cup brown lentils, rinsed
- 1 large potato, diced
- 3 tablespoons extra-virgin olive oil, plus more for drizzling
- 1 medium onion, coarsely chopped

- 1 teaspoon salt, divided
- Ground pepper to taste
- 1/2 bunch chard, coarsely chopped (about 2 cups)
- 1 lemon, cut into wedges

Instructions:

1. In a large pot, combine water and lentils. Bring to a high heat until simmering, then reduce to maintain a simmer. Stir occasionally and cook until lentils are almost tender, approximately 5 minutes. Add potato and continue cooking for an additional 10 minutes.

2. Meanwhile, in a medium skillet over medium heat, heat oil. Add onion, 1/2 teaspoon salt, and pepper to taste. Cook, stirring occasionally, until the onions turn golden brown, approximately 10 to 15 minutes. Adjust heat and add water by the tablespoon, if needed, to prevent burning.

3. Integrate the sautéed onion and chard into the simmering soup. Cook until the potato reaches tenderness, around 5 minutes more. Season with the remaining 1/2 teaspoon salt and additional pepper if desired. Serve the soup with lemon wedges.

Nutrition Facts (per serving): 376 Calories / 8g Fat / 70g Carbs / 14g Protein

Coconut Stew with Spinach & Beans

Infuse this stew with the sweet and hearty goodness of sweet potatoes, complemented by the flavors of ginger, cumin, coriander, and the vibrant yellow hue of turmeric. Unseeded chiles bring an extra kick, but you can mellow the spiciness by removing the seeds. The key is to cook the potatoes until tender, yet maintaining their shape, as the residual heat will continue to cook them after the stew is removed from heat.

Active Time: 40 mins
Total Time: 40 mins
Servings: 4 servings

Ingredients:
- 2 tablespoons extra-virgin olive oil
- 1 small yellow onion, chopped
- 2 tablespoons chopped unseeded jalapeño pepper
- 1 tablespoon finely chopped garlic
- 2 teaspoons finely chopped fresh ginger
- 2 tablespoons unsalted tomato paste
- 1 1/2 teaspoons ground cumin
- 1/2 teaspoon ground coriander
- 1/2 teaspoon ground turmeric
- 2 cups water
- 1 (13 1/2 ounce) can light coconut milk
- 1 pound scrubbed sweet potatoes, sliced crosswise 1/2-inch thick
- 1 (15-ounce) can no-salt-added cannellini beans, rinsed
- 1 (5-ounce) package fresh spinach
- 1/2 teaspoon salt
- 1 tablespoon lemon juice

Instructions:
1. Begin by heating oil in a large saucepan over medium-high heat. Sauté the onion until it starts to brown, approximately 6 minutes. Introduce jalapeño, garlic, and ginger, stirring often until fragrant (about 1 minute). Add tomato paste, cumin, coriander, and turmeric, stirring constantly until fragrant and the vegetables are well-coated (roughly 30 seconds).

2. Pour in water and coconut milk, bringing the mixture to a vigorous simmer over high heat. Reduce the heat to medium and introduce the sweet potatoes, allowing them to reach a gentle boil. Cook, stirring occasionally, until the sweet potatoes are tender, about 15 minutes.

3. Incorporate beans, spinach, and salt, stirring until the spinach wilts (approximately 1 minute). Remove the pot from heat and add a touch of freshness with a stir of lemon juice.

Nutrition Facts (per serving): 341 Calories / 14g Fat / 46g Carbs / 11g Protein

Cheeseburger Casserole

Indulge in the delightful flavors of a classic cheeseburger with a family-friendly twist in this Cheeseburger Casserole. Rotini pasta serves as the perfect canvas to absorb all the comforting goodness, but any pasta shape from your pantry will work just as well. While shredded fresh lettuce adds a satisfying crunch, don't hesitate to experiment with alternatives like spinach, kale, or elevate it with Swiss cheese and sautéed mushrooms for a unique spin.

Active Time: 30 mins
Total Time: 30 mins
Servings: 6 servings

Ingredients:
- 8 ounces whole-wheat rotini
- 1 tablespoon extra-virgin olive oil
- 1/2 cup chopped onion
- 1 pound lean ground beef
- 1 15-ounce can of no-salt-added petite diced tomatoes
- 2 tablespoons dill relish plus 1 teaspoon, divided
- 2 tablespoons ketchup, divided
- 1 tablespoon prepared yellow mustard
- 3/4 teaspoon salt
- 1/4 teaspoon ground pepper
- 1 cup shredded Cheddar cheese
- 3 tablespoons mayonnaise
- 1 1/2 cups shredded iceberg or romaine lettuce

Instructions:
1. Begin by bringing a large pot of water to a boil. Cook the rotini according to package instructions, then drain and set it aside.

2. In a spacious skillet over medium heat, heat oil. Sauté the onion until softened (about 3 minutes), then add the ground beef, cooking until it's no longer pink (approximately 7 minutes). Incorporate tomatoes with their juices, 2 tablespoons relish, 1 tablespoon ketchup, mustard, salt, and pepper. Bring the mixture to a simmer and cook, stirring, until the liquid reduces by half (around 3 minutes). Add the cooked rotini,

sprinkle with cheese, and remove from heat. Cover and let it stand until the cheese melts (approximately 5 minutes).

3. While the casserole rests, mix mayonnaise with the remaining 1 tablespoon of ketchup and 1 teaspoon of relish in a small bowl.

4. Serve the casserole with a sprinkle of lettuce and a drizzle of the sauce for a deliciously familiar yet uniquely crafted experience.

Nutrition Information: Serving Size: 1 1/3 cups
Calories 442, Fat 23g, Saturated Fat 8g, Cholesterol 71mg, Carbohydrates 35g, Total Sugars 5g, Added Sugars 1g, Protein 26g, Fiber 5g, Sodium 707mg, Potassium 488mg.

Ginger-Soy Salmon Balls

Elevate your dining experience with these delectable ginger-soy salmon balls. They stand out on their own, paired with your preferred starch and veggies, or add a protein punch to salads or grain bowls. Whether you opt for salmon packed in water or oil, make sure it's well-drained. Select boneless and skinless salmon for effortless rolling.

Active Time: 15 mins
Total Time: 35 mins
Servings: 4 servings

Ingredients:
- 2 6-ounce cans of boneless, skinless salmon, drained well
- 1/4 cup panko breadcrumbs, preferably whole-wheat
- 1 large scallion, chopped
- 1 large egg, lightly beaten
- 1 tablespoon mayonnaise
- 2 teaspoons grated fresh ginger
- 1 tablespoon reduced-sodium soy sauce

Instructions:
1. Begin by preheating the oven to 400°F and coating a large, rimmed baking sheet with cooking spray.

2. In a generous mixing bowl, combine salmon, panko, scallion, egg, mayonnaise, and ginger. Stir the ingredients, ensuring the salmon is well incorporated. With clean hands, shape the mixture into 16 balls, approximately 1½ tablespoons each, and arrange them on the prepared baking sheet. Bake, turning once, until the balls are firm and golden, taking about 20 minutes. Once out of the oven, drizzle the salmon balls with soy sauce, stirring gently to coat them thoroughly.

Nutrition Facts (per serving): 167 Calories / 8g Fat / 5g Carbs / 19g Protein

Easy Tofu Curry

Achieve optimal texture and shape retention for your protein-packed tofu curry by baking the tofu before incorporating it into the sauce. The curry itself boasts a smooth and creamy consistency, enriched with warmth from various spices and a hint of heat from Madras curry powder and jalapeño. To tone down the spice, you can switch Madras curry powder to regular curry powder. Tearing the tofu by hand ensures that the curry sauce adheres to all the intricate crevices, but if preferred, you can cut the tofu into 1-inch cubes instead.

Active Time: 30 mins
Total Time: 40 mins
Servings: 4 servings

Nutrition Notes:
Is Brown Basmati Rice Good for You?
Brown basmati rice, an aromatic whole grain, emanates a delightful nutty fragrance during cooking. Unlike white rice, which undergoes processing that removes nutritious outer layers, brown basmati rice retains valuable nutrients such as antioxidants, fiber, and plant-based protein.

Are Peas Healthy?
Peas, a versatile vegetable, offer significant health benefits. A cup of peas provides nearly a day's worth of vitamin C, along with a substantial boost of protein and fiber. Additionally, peas contain essential vitamins and minerals like iron, zinc, and B vitamins.

Is This Recipe Gluten-Free?
Despite its varied ingredients, this recipe is gluten-free, ensuring a wholesome dining experience for those with gluten sensitivities.

Tips from the Test Kitchen:
Why Should I Bake the Tofu Before Adding It to the Curry?
Baking the tofu beforehand enhances its shape retention in the curry. The addition of garam masala contributes an extra layer of flavor, while cornstarch crisps up the tofu, imparting a desirable texture.

How Can I Adjust the Spice Level of the Curry?
To lower the spice level, substitute Madras curry powder with regular curry powder. Madras curry powder tends to be spicier due to the inclusion of dried hot peppers in its blend.

Can I Make Tofu Curry Ahead?
Absolutely! Allow the curry to cool completely before refrigerating it in an airtight container, where it can be stored for up to 3 days.

Frequently Asked Questions:
What Kind of Tofu Should I Use in Curry?
For optimal structure during simmering, opt for extra-firm tofu. Softer variants like soft tofu or silken tofu, while creamy in texture, are less sturdy and may disintegrate in the curry. Save these for smoothies and desserts where their creaminess shines.

Ingredients:
- 1 (14-ounce) package extra-firm tofu, drained, pressed, and patted dry
- 3 tablespoons canola oil, divided
- 2 tablespoons cornstarch
- 1 1/2 teaspoons garam masala, divided
- 1 teaspoon salt, divided
- 1 cup chopped yellow onion
- 1 medium jalapeño pepper, stemmed and finely chopped
- 1 (1 1/2-inch) piece fresh ginger, peeled and finely chopped

- 4 cloves garlic, finely chopped
- 1 tablespoon Madras curry powder
- 1 (15-ounce) can no-salt-added crushed tomatoes
- 1 cup well-stirred canned coconut milk
- 1/2 cup water
- 1 (10-ounce) package frozen peas
- 1 (5-ounce) package baby spinach
- 2 cups hot cooked brown basmati rice
- Fresh cilantro leaves and tender stems for garnish (optional)

Instructions:

1. Preheat your oven to 400°F. Begin by using your hands to crumble tofu into bite-sized pieces onto a rimmed baking sheet. Gently toss the crumbled tofu with 2 tablespoons of oil, cornstarch, 1 teaspoon of garam masala, and 1/2 teaspoon of salt until the pieces are evenly coated. Bake the mixture, stirring once halfway through, until it achieves a light golden color with crispy edges, taking approximately 30 minutes.

2. While the tofu bakes, heat the remaining 1 tablespoon of oil in a medium Dutch oven over medium heat. Add onion, jalapeño, ginger, and garlic, cooking and stirring frequently until softened, which should take about 5 minutes. Incorporate curry powder, along with the remaining 1/2 teaspoon each of garam masala and salt. Stir constantly until the aroma becomes fragrant, about 30 seconds.

3. Introduce tomatoes and coconut milk to the Dutch oven, simmering the mixture over medium heat. Allow the flavors to meld for about 5 minutes.

4. Ladle the simmered mixture into a blender, securing the lid while leaving a gap for steam to escape. Cover the opening with a clean towel. Process the ingredients until the blend becomes smooth and creamy, taking approximately 1 minute. Exercise caution when blending hot liquids. Return the pureed mixture to the pot. Alternatively, use an immersion blender to achieve a smooth consistency directly in the pot, which should take about 2 minutes.

5. Add the baked tofu, water, peas, and spinach to the pot. Cook over medium heat, stirring occasionally, until the peas become tender and the spinach wilts, requiring 3 to 5 minutes.

6. Divide the rice among 4 bowls and top each with the prepared curry. Garnish with cilantro if desired, and enjoy the rich flavors of this aromatic and hearty dish.

Nutrition Facts (per serving): 555 Calories / 30g Fat / 59g Carbs / 22g Protein

Spicy Crispy Roasted Cauliflower

In her latest cookbook, Lidia Bastianich expresses her love for cauliflower and acknowledges that not everyone shares the same sentiment. To win over cauliflower skeptics, she shares a recipe that transforms this vegetable into crispy, bite-sized florets in the oven. These delightful morsels can be served as finger food for gatherings, appetizers, or as an additional vegetable for any meal. Originally created for her grandkids as a healthier alternative to typical fried finger foods, these crispy florets are a crowd-pleaser. Whether sprinkled with lemon juice or dipped in a favorite family sauce, they offer a delightful crunch. And, for an extra kick, ketchup with Calabrese peperoncino is recommended.

Active Time: 10 mins
Total Time: 35 mins

Ingredients:
- ¾ cup fine dry breadcrumbs
- ¾ cup freshly grated pecorino or Grana Padano, or a combination
- 1 teaspoon garlic powder
- 1 teaspoon onion powder
- 1 stick unsalted butter, melted
- 1 large head cauliflower, cut into florets
- ¼ teaspoon kosher salt
- Warm marinara for dipping (optional)

Instructions:
1. Preheat your oven to 425 degrees F and line two baking sheets with parchment paper.

2. In a large bowl, combine breadcrumbs, cheese, garlic powder, and onion powder. In another large bowl, melt butter and add cauliflower. Season with salt and toss to coat the cauliflower in butter. Take half of the cauliflower and toss it in the breadcrumb mixture until thoroughly coated. Place the coated cauliflower on one of the prepared baking sheets. Repeat this process with the remaining cauliflower and breadcrumbs, discarding any unused breadcrumbs.

3. Bake the cauliflower in the preheated oven until it achieves a deep golden brown and crispy texture, typically taking 25 to 30 minutes. Serve the warm, crispy cauliflower with marinara for dipping, if desired. Enjoy this flavorful and versatile cauliflower dish that turns skeptics into fans.

Nutrition Facts (per serving): 235 Calories / 18g Fat / 13g Carbs / 7g Protein

Bibimbap-Inspired Rice Bowls

Though not following tradition precisely, these brown rice bowls pack a protein punch and draw inspiration from Korean bibimbap. The dish features a delightful combination of sweet and spicy ground beef, sliced veggies, and a crowning touch—a perfectly fried egg. Gochujang, a fermented paste crafted from chiles, soybeans, and rice, lends a nuanced spiciness and a myriad of flavors. The dish is completed with the addition of toasted sesame oil, imparting a delightful nuttiness.

Active Time: 30 mins
Total Time: 30 mins
Servings: 4

Ingredients:
- 2 tablespoons reduced-sodium soy sauce
- 1 tablespoon gochujang
- 1 tablespoon rice vinegar
- 1 tablespoon honey
- 1 teaspoon sesame oil
- 1 teaspoon grated garlic
- 3 small scallions
- 2 tablespoons canola oil, divided
- 1 cup chopped white onion

- 1 pound lean ground beef
- ¼ teaspoon salt
- 4 large eggs
- 2 cups hot cooked brown rice
- 2 small Persian cucumbers, thinly sliced
- 1 cup matchstick carrots
- 1 cup thinly sliced radish
- 1 tablespoon toasted sesame seeds
- 1 ½ tablespoons toasted sesame oil

Instructions:

1. In a small bowl, combine soy sauce, gochujang, vinegar, honey, sesame oil, and garlic. Slice the white and light green parts of the scallions at a 1/4-inch angle, totaling around 1/4 cup. Additionally, thinly slice the dark green scallion parts at an angle, amounting to about 2 tablespoons.

2. Heat 1 tablespoon of canola oil in a wok or large nonstick skillet over medium-high heat until shimmering. Sauté the onion, stirring often, until softened and translucent, roughly 4 minutes. Add ground beef and salt, continuously stirring to break the meat into crumbles. Cook until browned, approximately 4 to 5 minutes. Introduce the soy sauce mixture and stir often until the sauce slightly thickens and coats the meat, approximately 2 minutes. Stir in the white and light green scallion slices. Remove from heat and cover.

3. In a separate large nonstick skillet, heat the remaining 1 tablespoon of canola oil over medium-high heat. Crack eggs into the pan and cook until the whites are set with crispy edges, taking about 3 minutes. Remove from heat.

4. Divide the rice evenly among 4 bowls. Top each with the beef mixture, cucumbers, carrots, radishes, and a fried egg. Sprinkle the dark green scallion slices and sesame seeds over each bowl. Drizzle toasted sesame oil evenly for the finishing touch. Enjoy the rich flavors and diverse textures of these inspired brown rice bowls.

Nutrition Facts (per serving): 599 Calories / 32g Fat / 44g Carbs / 34g Protein

Pasta alla Norma

Sicilian-inspired, our take on Pasta alla Norma combines eggplant, tomatoes, and ricotta salata. While retaining the essence of the traditional dish, we infuse a touch of sweetness and flavor with balsamic vinegar and fennel seeds. Ricotta salata, a firm, salty cheese, along with basil, adds vibrancy to this effortlessly prepared vegetarian delight.

Active Time: 50 mins
Total Time: 55 mins
Servings: 8

Nutrition Notes:
For a gluten-free option, substitute whole-wheat rigatoni with gluten-free rigatoni or another gluten-free pasta. Alternatively, serve the eggplant mixture over polenta, a naturally gluten-free choice. Use store-bought polenta or try our Creamy Polenta recipe for a tasty variation.

Do You Need to Salt the Eggplant Before Cooking? While many recipes advise salting eggplant before cooking to preserve its firmness and prevent mushiness, we avoid this step to limit sodium intake. The dish remains delicious without salting the eggplant.

Tips from the Test Kitchen: Ricotta Salata Substitute: If ricotta salata is unavailable, consider feta, Pecorino Romano, or cotija cheese as suitable alternatives. Each provides a mild and salty flavor akin to ricotta salata.

Storing Leftovers: To maintain pasta texture, store the sauce and cooked pasta separately in airtight containers for up to 4 days. Reheat on the stovetop or in the microwave until warm.

Frequently Asked Questions:
Where Does Pasta Alla Norma Come From? Originating in Catania, Sicily, Pasta alla Norma draws its name from Vincenzo Bellini's opera Norma. Nino Martoglio, upon tasting it, exclaimed it as a culinary masterpiece, dubbing it a "real Norma."

Ingredients:
- 2 large eggplants (about 21 ounces each) unpeeled and cubed (1-inch)
- 4 tablespoons extra-virgin olive oil, divided
- 2 tablespoons balsamic vinegar
- 8 medium cloves garlic, chopped
- 1 tablespoon tomato paste
- 1 (28-ounce) can no-salt-added whole peeled plum tomatoes, undrained
- 1 large basil sprig, plus basil leaves for garnish
- ¾ teaspoon fennel seeds
- ¾ teaspoon salt
- ¼ teaspoon crushed red pepper
- 1 pound whole-wheat rigatoni
- 6 tablespoons crumbled ricotta salata cheese

Instructions:
1. Preheat the oven to 375°F and line two baking sheets with parchment paper.
2. Toss eggplant with oil and vinegar; spread on baking sheets. Bake until golden and tender, stirring and rotating pans halfway through.
3. In a Dutch oven, sauté garlic, add tomato paste, then tomatoes, basil, fennel seeds, salt, and crushed red pepper. Simmer until thickened.
4. Cook pasta until al dente; reserve 1/2 cup cooking water.
5. Stir baked eggplant into the tomato sauce, add pasta and reserved water. Coat evenly.
6. Divide among bowls, top with ricotta salata, and garnish with basil leaves if desired.

Equipment: Parchment paper
Nutrition Facts (per serving): 336 Calories / 10g Fat / 52g Carbs / 11g Protein

Lemony-Garlic Pan-Seared Salmon

This pan-seared salmon showcases a medley of fresh herbs, zesty lemon, and savory garlic. Opting to leave the skin on not only preserves the fillet's integrity during cooking but also yields delightfully crispy skin that can be effortlessly removed if a skinless preference exists.

Active Time: 15 mins
Total Time: 15 mins
Servings: 4

Ingredients:
- 4 (5-ounce) skin-on salmon fillets
- ½ teaspoon garlic powder
- ½ teaspoon salt
- ½ teaspoon salt-free lemon pepper
- 1 tablespoon extra-virgin olive oil
- 1 large clove garlic, crushed
- 1 tablespoon unsalted butter
- 1 tablespoon chopped fresh herbs, such as parsley, chives and/or dill
- ½ teaspoon grated lemon zest
- Lemon wedges for serving

Nutrition Notes:
Is Salmon Healthy? Absolutely! Salmon, a fatty fish, is abundant in heart-healthy omega-3 fatty acids known for reducing inflammation, lowering triglyceride levels, blood pressure, blood clot risks, and irregular heartbeats. The presence of the antioxidant astaxanthin, responsible for the fish's orange hue, further fortifies salmon against inflammation, benefiting cardiovascular health, cancer prevention, eye health, and anti-aging.

Is It Safe to Eat Salmon Skin? Yes, salmon skin is safe to consume and boasts the same nutrients as the flesh. Keeping the skin on post-cooking enhances the retention of healthy fats and nutrients.

What Are the Nutritional Differences Between Wild and Farmed Salmon? While wild salmon tends to have lower fat content due to increased exercise in foraging, both wild and farmed options offer heart-healthy fats. Wild salmon's deeper-colored flesh indicates higher astaxanthin levels. Choose based on preference, considering potential differences in taste and cooking characteristics.

Tips from the Test Kitchen:
Is Salmon Sustainable? Ensure sustainable choices by considering factors like salmon type, origin, and catch method. Reputable sources like Seafood Watch or the Marine Stewardship Council provide updated information on sustainable options.

No Lemon Pepper? Substitute your preferred salt-free seasoning or create a homemade Salmon Seasoning.

Buying the Freshest Salmon: Select firm fillets that rebound to the touch, emit a mild, neutral scent, and lack an overly fishy odor.

I Bought Skinless Salmon—No Recipe Adjustment Needed: Follow the recipe as is; pan-sear skinless salmon fillets according to Step 2.

Frequently Asked Questions:
What Side of Salmon Do You Sear First? Begin by searing the salmon skin-side down for 3 to 4 minutes until crisp, then flip.

No Thermometer? Look for Opaque and Flakey: While an instant-read thermometer is ideal, observe opaque flesh and easy flaking with a fork to determine doneness.

Instructions:
1. Pat salmon dry, season with garlic powder, salt, and lemon pepper.

2. Heat oil in a nonstick skillet, sear salmon skin-side down until crisp. 3. Flip, add garlic and butter, cook until the internal temperature reaches 145°F.
4. Transfer salmon to a platter, and sprinkle with herbs and lemon zest. Serve with lemon wedges.

Nutrition Facts (per serving): 259 Calories / 15g Fat / 1g Carbs / 28g Protein

HEALTHY HIGH-BLOOD PRESSURE RECIPES

Chipotle Chicken Quinoa Burrito Bowl

This flavorful burrito bowl showcases grilled chicken coated in a zesty chipotle glaze, elevating its taste. Packed with nutritious elements such as quinoa instead of rice and an assortment of vegetables, it transforms into a wholesome dinner option.

Active Time: 30 mins
Total Time: 30 mins
Servings: 4
Yield: 4 burrito bowls

Ingredients:
- 1 tablespoon finely chopped chipotle peppers in adobo sauce
- 1 tablespoon extra-virgin olive oil
- ½ teaspoon garlic powder
- ½ teaspoon ground cumin
- 1 pound boneless, skinless chicken breast
- ¼ teaspoon salt
- 2 cups cooked quinoa
- 2 cups shredded romaine lettuce
- 1 cup canned pinto beans, rinsed
- 1 ripe avocado, diced
- ¼ cup prepared pico de gallo or other salsa
- ¼ cup shredded Cheddar or Monterey Jack cheese
- Lime wedges for serving

Instructions:
1. Preheat the grill to medium-high or preheat the broiler.

2. In a small bowl, combine chipotle, oil, garlic powder, and cumin.

3. If grilling, oil the grill rack (refer to Tip) or, for broiling, use a rimmed baking sheet. Season the chicken with salt. Grill the chicken for 5 minutes or broil it on the prepared baking sheet for 9 minutes.

4. Turn the chicken, brush it with the chipotle glaze, and continue cooking until an instant-read thermometer inserted in the thickest part registers 165 degrees F, taking an additional 3 to 5 minutes on the grill or 9 minutes under the broiler. Transfer the cooked chicken to a clean cutting board and chop it into bite-size pieces.

5. Assemble each burrito bowl with 1/2 cup quinoa, 1/2 cup grilled chicken, 1/2 cup lettuce, 1/4 cup beans, 1/4 avocado, 1 tablespoon pico de gallo (or an alternative salsa), and 1 tablespoon cheese.

6. Serve each bowl with a lime wedge for added flavor.

Tips: To oil a grill rack, oil a folded paper towel, hold it with tongs and rub it over the rack. (Do not use cooking spray on a hot grill.)
Nutrition Facts (per serving): 452 Calories / 19g Fat / 36g Carbs / 36g Protein

Mushroom-Swiss Turkey Burgers

In this gluten-free turkey burger recipe, lean ground turkey replaces ground beef, and portobello mushrooms serve as a juicy, flavorful substitute for the traditional bun. Topped with melted Swiss cheese, sliced tomato, and arugula, this delightful low-carb dinner is both delicious and satisfying!

Prep Time: 20 mins
Additional Time: 10 mins
Total Time: 30 mins
Servings: 4
Yield: 4 burgers

Ingredients:
- 2 tablespoons extra-virgin olive oil
- 1 clove garlic, minced
- ¾ teaspoon ground pepper, divided
- ½ teaspoon salt, divided
- 8 portobello mushroom caps, stems and gills removed (see Tips)
- 1 pound lean ground turkey
- 2 teaspoons gluten-free Worcestershire sauce
- 1 teaspoon Dijon mustard
- 4 slices Swiss cheese
- 1 small tomato, thinly sliced
- 3 cups baby arugula

Instructions:
1. Preheat the grill to medium-high (400-450 degrees F). In a small bowl, mix oil, garlic, and 1/4 teaspoon each of pepper and salt. Brush the portobello caps with the oil mixture and let them marinate at room temperature for 10 minutes.

2. In a medium bowl, combine ground turkey, Worcestershire, mustard, and the remaining 1/2 teaspoon pepper and 1/4 teaspoon salt. Gently incorporate the ingredients without overmixing. Shape the mixture into four 3/4-inch-thick patties and set them aside.

3. Oil the grill rack (refer to Tips). Place the portobello caps, cap-side down, on the oiled grill rack. Grill, covered, until just tender, about 4 minutes per side. Transfer the mushrooms to a plate and cover to keep warm. Oil the rack again and place the turkey patties on the oiled rack. Grill, covered, until the patties are lightly charred and an instant-read thermometer inserted in the center registers 165 degrees F, approximately 4 to 5 minutes per side. Add a slice of cheese to each patty during the last minute of cooking. Transfer the patties to a plate and let them rest for 5 minutes. If your grill is large enough, you can grill the portobello caps and the patties simultaneously.

4. Place each turkey patty on the stem side of a portobello cap; top them evenly with tomato slices and arugula. Cover with the remaining portobello caps, stem-side down, and serve immediately.

Tips: To prepare portobello mushroom caps, gently twist off the stems of whole portobellos. Use a spoon to scrape off the brown gills from the underside of the mushroom caps. Alternatively, you can purchase portobello mushroom caps instead of whole mushrooms.
Oil the grill rack before grilling to prevent sticking. Use tongs to hold a folded paper towel dipped in vegetable oil, rubbing it over the rack (avoid using cooking spray on a hot grill).

Nutrition Facts (per serving): 332 Calories / 18g Fat / 10g Carbs / 34g Protein

Cheeseburger Stuffed Baked Potatoes

Ditch the bun and present a delectable alternative to the classic cheeseburger by pairing beef, cheese, tomatoes, red onions, and lettuce with baked potatoes. This hearty and straightforward dinner recipe is sure to be a hit with both kids and adults alike. Feel free to switch out the ground beef for ground turkey or tofu crumbles for a customized touch.

Prep Time: 10 mins
Additional Time: 15 mins
Total Time: 25 mins
Servings: 4
Yield: 4 potatoes

Ingredients:
- 4 medium russet potatoes (about 8 ounces each)
- ½ cup low-fat mayonnaise
- 8 ounces of cooked ground beef, warmed
- ½ cup shredded iceberg lettuce
- ½ cup diced tomato
- ¼ cup sliced red onion
- 4 teaspoons shredded Colby Jack cheese

Instructions:
1. Pierce potatoes all over with a fork. Microwave on Medium, turning once or twice, until soft, approximately 20 minutes. Alternatively, bake potatoes at 425 degrees F until tender, for 45 minutes to 1 hour. Transfer to a clean cutting board and allow them to cool slightly.

2. Safeguarding your hands with a kitchen towel, make a lengthwise cut to open the potato, ensuring not to cut all the way through. Pinch the ends to reveal the flesh.

3. Top each potato with a layer of mayonnaise, followed by beef, lettuce, tomato, red onion, and cheese. Serve while warm.

Nutrition Facts (per serving): 351 Calories / 11g Fat / 43g Carbs / 20g Protein

Vegan Smoothie Bowl

Savor this rich and velvety smoothie bowl with a spoon! Blend together banana, frozen berries, and a touch of nut milk for a delicious vegan breakfast base. Get creative with toppings—use a mix of fruits, nuts, and seeds, or explore your own favorite combinations.

Prep Time: 10 mins

Total Time: 10 mins
Servings: 1
Yield: 1 serving

Ingredients:
- 1 large banana
- 1 cup frozen mixed berries
- ½ cup unsweetened soymilk or other unsweetened non-dairy milk
- ¼ cup pineapple chunks
- ½ kiwi, sliced
- 1 tablespoon sliced almonds, toasted if desired
- 1 tablespoon unsweetened coconut flakes, toasted if desired
- 1 teaspoon chia seeds

Instructions:
1. In a blender, combine banana, berries, and soymilk (or almond milk). Blend until smooth.
2. Pour the smoothie into a bowl and embellish it with pineapple, kiwi, almonds, coconut, and chia seeds.

Nutrition Facts (per serving): 338 Calories / 10g Fat / 64g Carbs / 9g Protein

Baked Eggs with Roasted Vegetables

Packed with 11 grams of protein per serving, this breakfast recipe is ideal for a hearty start to the day. Save time by preparing it the night before and letting it chill overnight, requiring minimal effort in the morning.

Prep Time: 25 mins
Additional Time: 9 hrs
Total Time: 9 hrs 25 mins
Servings: 6
Yield: 6 servings

Ingredients:
- 3 cups small broccoli florets (about 1 inch in size)
- 12 ounces yellow potatoes, such as Yukon Gold, cut into 1/2- to 3/4-inch pieces (about 2 cups)
- 1 large sweet potato, cut into 1/2- to 3/4-inch pieces (about 1 cup)
- 1 small red onion, cut into thin slices
- 2 tablespoons olive oil
- 6 eggs
- 2 ounces Manchego cheese, shredded (1/2 cup)
- ½ teaspoon cracked black pepper

Instructions:
1. Preheat the oven to 425 degrees Fahrenheit. Grease a 2-quart rectangular baking dish with nonstick cooking spray. In a large bowl, toss broccoli, yellow potatoes, sweet potato, onion, olive oil, and 1/4 teaspoon salt until vegetables are evenly coated.

2. Spread the vegetable mixture evenly in the prepared pan. Roast for 10 minutes. Stir the vegetables and roast for an additional 5 minutes or until they are tender and starting to brown. Remove from the oven, spread the vegetables evenly in the baking dish, and let them cool. Cover and refrigerate for 8 to 24 hours.

3. Allow the chilled vegetables to stand at room temperature for 30 minutes. Meanwhile, preheat the oven to 375 degrees Fahrenheit.

4. Bake the vegetables, uncovered, for 5 minutes. Remove from the oven and create six wells in the vegetable layer. Crack one egg into each well. Bake for an additional 5 minutes. Sprinkle with cheese and bake for 5 to 10 minutes more or until the egg whites are set and the yolks are beginning to thicken. Season with pepper to taste.

Nutrition Facts (per serving): 232 Calories / 12g Fat / 21g Carbs / 11g Protein

Summer Skillet Vegetable & Egg Scramble

Don't discard those nearly overripe vegetables and fresh herbs—incorporate them into this speedy vegetarian skillet egg scramble. This versatile skillet recipe accommodates almost any vegetable, so feel free to pick your favorites or utilize what's available.

Prep Time: 30 mins
Total Time: 30 mins
Servings: 4
Yield: 6 cups

Ingredients:
- 2 tablespoons olive oil
- 12 ounces baby potatoes, thinly sliced
- 4 cups thinly sliced vegetables, such as mushrooms, bell peppers, and/or zucchini (14 oz.)
- 3 scallions, thinly sliced, green and white parts separated
- 1 teaspoon minced fresh herbs, such as rosemary or thyme
- 6 large eggs (or 4 large eggs plus 4 egg whites), lightly beaten
- 2 cups packed leafy greens, such as baby spinach or baby kale (2 oz.)
- ½ teaspoon salt

Instructions:
1. Heat oil in a generously sized cast-iron or nonstick skillet over medium heat. Add potatoes and cover, stirring occasionally, until they start to soften, approximately 8 minutes.

2. Introduce sliced vegetables and scallion whites; cook uncovered, stirring occasionally, until the vegetables achieve tenderness and a gentle browning, lasting 8 to 10 minutes. Mix in the herbs and push the vegetable blend to the edges of the pan.

3. Reduce the heat to medium-low. Incorporate eggs and scallion greens at the center of the pan. Stir continuously until the eggs form soft scrambles, taking around 2 minutes.

4. Integrate leafy greens into the eggs. Remove from heat and stir thoroughly to combine. Sprinkle in salt to taste.

Nutrition Facts (per serving): 254 Calories / 14g Fat / 20g Carbs / 12g Protein

English Muffin Pizza with Tomato & Olives

Transform your English muffin into a pizza-inspired delight, adorned with tomato, cheese, olives, and oregano. This versatile treat serves triple duty, making it an excellent snack, breakfast addition, or lunch feature.

Active Time: 5 mins
Total Time: 10 mins
Servings: 1

Ingredients:
- 1 whole-wheat English muffin, split and toasted
- 1 medium tomato, sliced
- 1 tablespoon sliced green olives
- 2 tablespoons shredded mozzarella cheese
- ⅛ teaspoon dried oregano

Instructions:
1. Preheat the broiler to high.

2. Distribute half of the tomato slices, olives, cheese, and oregano onto each English muffin half.
3. Broil for about 2 minutes, or until the cheese is melted and bubbly.

Nutrition Facts (per serving): 213 Calories / 5g Fat / 35g Carbs / 11g Protein

Walnut-Rosemary Crusted Salmon

Salmon and walnuts, both rich in omega-3 fatty acids, come together in this simple walnut-crusted salmon recipe. Create a wholesome dinner by pairing it with a straightforward salad and a side of roasted potatoes.

Cook Time: 10 mins
Active Time: 10 mins
Total Time: 20 mins
Servings: 4
Yield: 4 servings

Nutrition Notes:
Why is This Recipe Healthy? Every ingredient in this recipe contributes to its nutritional value. The salmon, the star of the dish, provides a substantial amount of protein—almost half of your daily requirement in one serving. Wild-caught salmon offers more than a day's worth of vitamin B12 and about three-quarters of your daily selenium, an antioxidant mineral. Salmon is also abundant in antioxidants like astaxanthin, known for its anti-inflammatory properties. Sockeye salmon, in particular, offers a significant dose of vitamin D—roughly 70% of your daily needs. Additionally, salmon is a rich source of heart-healthy omega-3 fatty acids.

How Can I Make This Recipe Gluten-Free? Swap the panko breadcrumbs with gluten-free panko breadcrumbs to create a gluten-free version of this dish.

Tips from the Test Kitchen:
Can I Use Dried Rosemary Instead of Fresh? Yes, you can substitute 1/4 to 1/2 teaspoon of dried rosemary for fresh rosemary.

Nut Allergy Substitute: If you have a nut allergy, finely chopped unsalted pumpkin seeds or sunflower seeds make an excellent alternative. Alternatively, omit the walnuts and increase the panko breadcrumbs by an additional 3 tablespoons.

What to Serve with Walnut-Rosemary Crusted Salmon:
This delightful walnut-crusted salmon complements well with simple vegetable side dishes like Roasted Asparagus, Roasted Broccoli, Crispy Oven-Roasted Potatoes, or Roasted Sweet Potatoes. Pair it with Brown Rice Pilaf, Creamy Cacio e Pepe Orzo, Whole-Wheat Couscous with Parmesan & Peas, or Mushroom Rice, and complete the meal with a simple green salad.

Ingredients:
- 2 teaspoons Dijon mustard
- 1 clove garlic, minced
- ¼ teaspoon lemon zest
- 1 teaspoon lemon juice
- 1 teaspoon chopped fresh rosemary
- ½ teaspoon honey
- ½ teaspoon kosher salt
- ¼ teaspoon crushed red pepper
- 3 tablespoons panko breadcrumbs
- 3 tablespoons finely chopped walnuts
- 1 teaspoon extra-virgin olive oil
- 1 (1 pound) skinless salmon fillet, fresh or frozen
- Olive oil cooking spray
- Chopped fresh parsley and lemon wedges for garnish

Instructions:
1. Preheat the oven to 425 degrees F and line a large-rimmed baking sheet with parchment paper.

2. In a small bowl, combine mustard, garlic, lemon zest, lemon juice, rosemary, honey, salt, and crushed red pepper.

3. In another small bowl, mix panko, walnuts, and oil.

4. Place the salmon on the prepared baking sheet. Spread the mustard mixture over the fish and sprinkle with the panko mixture, pressing it to adhere. Lightly coat with cooking spray.

5. Bake until the fish flakes easily with a fork, approximately 8 to 12 minutes, depending on thickness.

6. Sprinkle with parsley and serve with lemon wedges, if desired.

Equipment: Large rimmed baking sheet
Nutrition Facts (per serving): 222 Calories / 12g Fat / 4g Carbs / 24g Protein

Chickpea & Quinoa Grain Bowl

Grain bowls come in countless variations, much like the stars in the sky, and there's no incorrect method to assemble one! However, our inclination is towards the timeless and straightforward, featuring hummus, quinoa, avocado, and an abundance of veggies.

Prep Time: 15 mins
Total Time: 15 mins
Servings: 1
Yield: 1 serving

Ingredients:
- 1 cup cooked quinoa
- ⅓ cup canned chickpeas, rinsed and drained
- ½ cup cucumber slices
- ½ cup cherry tomatoes, halved
- ¼ avocado, diced
- 3 tablespoons hummus
- 1 tablespoon finely chopped roasted red pepper
- 1 tablespoon lemon juice
- 1 tablespoon water, plus more if desired
- 1 teaspoon chopped fresh parsley (Optional)
- Pinch of salt
- Pinch of ground pepper

Instructions:
1. In a wide bowl, arrange quinoa, chickpeas, cucumbers, tomatoes, and avocado.
2. In a separate bowl, mix hummus, roasted red pepper, lemon juice, and water. Adjust the water quantity to achieve the desired dressing consistency. Introduce parsley, salt, and pepper, stirring to blend. Serve alongside the Buddha bowl.

Nutrition Facts (per serving): 503 Calories / 17g Fat / 75g Carbs / 18g Protein

Maple-Roasted Chicken Thighs with Sweet Potato Wedges and Brussels Sprouts

This simple sheet-pan recipe brings together a medley of fall favorites for a satisfying dinner.

Prep Time: 20 mins
Additional Time: 30 mins
Total Time: 50 mins
Servings: 4
Yield: 4 servings

Ingredients:
- 2 tablespoons pure maple syrup
- 4 teaspoons olive oil
- 1 tablespoon snipped fresh thyme
- ½ teaspoon salt
- ½ teaspoon black pepper
- 1 pound sweet potatoes, peeled and cut into 1-inch wedges
- 1 pound Brussels sprouts, trimmed and halved
- Nonstick cooking spray
- 4 bone-in chicken thighs, skinned
- 3 tablespoons snipped dried cranberries
- 3 tablespoons chopped pecans, toasted

Instructions:

1. Preheat the oven to 425 degrees F. In a small bowl, combine maple syrup, 1 tsp. of oil, thyme, 1/4 tsp. salt, and 1/4 tsp. pepper.

2. In a large bowl, toss sweet potatoes and Brussels sprouts with the remaining 1 tbsp. oil, and sprinkle with the remaining 1/4 tsp. salt and 1/4 tsp. pepper; ensure the vegetables are evenly coated.

3. Line a 15x10-inch baking pan with foil. Heat the pan in the oven for 5 minutes. Remove and coat with cooking spray.

4. Arrange chicken, meaty sides down, in the center of the pan. Surround the chicken with the prepared vegetables. Roast for 15 minutes.

5. Turn the chicken and vegetables; brush them with the maple syrup mixture. Continue roasting for an additional 15 minutes or until the chicken reaches a minimum internal temperature of 175 degrees F, and the potatoes are tender.

6. Serve the dish topped with pecans and cranberries.

Nutrition Facts (per serving): 436 Calories / 14g Fat / 45g Carbs / 34g Protein

Summer Skillet Vegetable & Egg Scramble

Utilize those vegetables and fresh herbs that are nearly past their prime by incorporating them into this speedy skillet egg scramble, offering a swift and flavorful vegetarian meal. This uncomplicated skillet recipe accommodates a wide range of vegetables, so feel free to pick your favorites or make use of what's available.

Prep Time: 30 mins
Total Time: 30 mins
Servings: 4
Yield: 6 cups

Ingredients:
- 2 tablespoons olive oil
- 12 ounces baby potatoes, thinly sliced
- 4 cups thinly sliced vegetables, such as mushrooms, bell peppers, and/or zucchini (14 oz.)
- 3 scallions, thinly sliced, green and white parts separated
- 1 teaspoon minced fresh herbs, such as rosemary or thyme
- 6 large eggs (or 4 large eggs plus 4 egg whites), lightly beaten
- 2 cups packed leafy greens, such as baby spinach or baby kale (2 oz.)
- ½ teaspoon salt

Instructions:

1. Heat oil in a large cast-iron or nonstick skillet over medium heat. Add potatoes, cover, and cook, stirring occasionally, until they start to soften, approximately 8 minutes.

2. Introduce sliced vegetables and scallion whites; cook uncovered, stirring occasionally, until the vegetables become tender and lightly browned, lasting 8 to 10 minutes. Blend in the herbs, then shift the vegetable mixture to the perimeter of the pan.

3. Reduce the heat to medium-low. Add eggs and scallion greens to the center of the pan. Cook, stirring, until the eggs form soft scrambles, taking around 2 minutes.

4. Incorporate leafy greens into the eggs. Remove from heat and stir thoroughly to combine. Season with salt to taste.

Nutrition Facts (per serving): 254 Calories / 14g Fat / 20g Carbs / 12g Protein

Thank you!

We are constantly striving to provide the ideal experience for the community, and your input helps us to define that experience. So we kindly ask you when you have free time take a minute to post a review on Amazon.

Thank you for helping us support our passions.

TO LEAVE A REVIEW, JUST SCAN THE QR CODE BELOW:

OR YOU CAN GO TO:

amazon.com/review/create-review/

Made in the USA
Las Vegas, NV
24 September 2024

95751284R00090